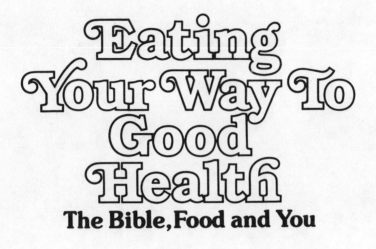

Eating Your Way To Good Health

The Bible, Food and You

Jean G. Wade
and
Helen Kooiman Hosier

Fleming H. Revell Company
Old Tappan, New Jersey

Library of Congress Cataloging in Publication Data

Wade, Jean G
    Eating your way to good health.

    Bibliography: p.
    1. Nutrition. 2. Food in the Bible. 3. Cookery.
I. Hosier, Helen Kooiman, joint author. II. Title.
RA784.W274   641.1   77-11898
ISBN 0-8007-0892-X

Contents

Preface

What is God's will for us in the area of food? Are there guidelines in the Bible which will help us choose food wisely, so that people of today can have better physical health?

We believe that there are, and our purpose is to seek out those guidelines, that they may be applied today. The Lord said: ". . . when ye did eat, and when ye did drink, did not ye eat for yourselves, and drink for yourselves?" (Zechariah 7:6 KJV). These words clearly indicate that people (and this applies to many Christians today) eat and drink for their own pleasure, and not in a manner which would strengthen their bodies and improve their health, so that they could better serve the Lord.

As a nutritionist working with various government agencies, I have observed that much ill health among individuals is due to the eating of foods which do not adequately nourish their bodies. People often are not aware that they are eating an inadequate diet because of a lack of knowledge about what constitutes good nutrition. This book is written to bring information and hope to people who desire a better understanding of how our bodies work and how health may be maintained by better dietary practices. We should ever keep in mind the admonition: "Whether therefore ye eat, or drink, or whatsoever ye do, do all to the glory of God" (1 Corinthians 10:31 KJV).

JEAN G. WADE

Introduction

For many years I was in the Christian bookselling business. There I observed a great hunger on the part of many for spiritual food. Some were less likely to seek out this form of spiritual nourishment. I often used a little maxim to show people the value of choosing their reading diet wisely. Individuals and audiences heard me say over and over again, "Next year you will be the same person you are today, except for the friends you make, the books you read, and the food you eat."

I was concerned about the reading habits of the people I encountered. I used that little saying to motivate them to read more often and to be very selective about what they were feeding their minds—the nourishment that was needed for what we refer to as the inner man (the spirit).

Now I am fulfilling a longtime desire, something that has become a conviction based on my own experiences, observations of what is happening to others, and extensive reading and long hours of study. When Jean Wade's manuscript came to my attention I recognized in her a kindred spirit. She had done what I knew needed doing and what I intended some day to do. Now I can use my favorite maxim and emphasize the latter part.

Both Jean and I are convinced of the need for responsible stewardship of our bodies, the temples of the Holy Spirit. We believe it is our responsibility to cooperate with our all-wise Creator in caring for these earthly temples.

One young woman who had shown an interest in my work said, "Mrs. Hosier, I do believe you are a food faddist." If it is being a food faddist to deeply care for the physical well-being (as well as the spiritual well-being) of others, then both Jean and I gladly accept the label.

Eating your way to good health can be a joy-filled daily experience. This is our desire for you and those you love.

HELEN HOSIER

1

In the Beginning . . .

Then the Lord God planted a garden . . .
Genesis 2:8

After hearing the Creation account from her favorite Bible storybook a little girl asked her mother, "Mom, how did God get the dust in us?"

There are those who reject the Genesis story of Creation, but like that trusting child, we choose to believe it. It seems altogether reasonable that if a person believes in this, he also accepts the fact that since man was created from the dust of the ground (Genesis 2:7), it is in mankind's best interests to look to the ground and what it contains and produces to sustain his life. If the all-wise Creator made the first man from the ground, then obviously all the elements in the soil necessary for the building of a body were there to begin with. God in His infinite wisdom neglected nothing.

When God Planted a Garden

The first man had no way of knowing how to care for his body. At the very outset of Creation, therefore, God made provision for His created beings to survive. ". . . look!" he said, "I have given you the seed-bearing plants throughout the earth, and all the fruit trees for your food" (Genesis 1:29).

God planned in the very beginning that fruits and vegetables should form a large part of man's diet. We have neglected these elemental instructions from our Creator to our own detriment. How far we have strayed from the Creator's plan!

God told Adam that He was placing him in the Garden of Eden so that he could dress the trees and tend to that which grew there (Genesis 2:15). When God spoke into being the matchless wonders of the sun, moon, stars, planets, galaxies, plants, and moving creatures, and man himself, we are repeatedly told that "God saw that it was good."

God established perfect law and order in the system of nature. When we violate these, we have to suffer the consequences. Adam was told what to do, and God hasn't altered the order of growing things.

The prohibition which God placed upon Adam and Eve shows the importance that God attached to food.

> The Lord God planted all sorts of beautiful trees there in the garden, trees producing the choicest of fruit. At the center of the garden he placed the Tree of Life, and also the Tree of Conscience, giving knowledge of Good and Bad. A river from the land of Eden flowed through the garden to water it . . .
>
> The Lord God placed the man in the Garden of Eden as its gardener, to tend and care for it. But the Lord God gave the man this warning: "You may eat any fruit in the garden except fruit from the Tree of Conscience—for its fruit will open your eyes to make you aware of right and wrong, good and bad. If you eat its fruit, you will be doomed to die."
>
> Genesis 2:9, 10, 15–17

This was a "No-no," but the world's first gardener failed the test.

Eve, You Did It!

Women, for the most part, are responsible for the feeding and nourishment of their husbands and children, and ever since that incident, they have been getting the human race into trouble by setting the wrong food before their families. This is not intended as a blanket indictment against all women, for some, indeed, have learned to obey the biblical rules for good nutrition. It is necessary to recognize that as wives and mothers we are accountable for what our families eat.

Tempted by Food

Eve's ready availability to lend an ear to what the serpent was saying cost her, and every human being since then, ruin, disfigurement, and death. The serpent's deception struck at man's weakest point at the very outset of man's life upon planet earth. We've been reaping the results of that weakness in every generation since the garden encounter. Tempted by food, we bring about many of our own physical troubles. It would seem that our Creator was trying to get a message across to us from the beginning—the message that food could bring about our downfall in more ways than one. How slow we are to learn!

Why Weeds?

Man's craving for forbidden food resulted in God placing a curse upon the soil. All his life, man would struggle to extract a living from it (Genesis 3:17–19). This is the first biblically recorded instance of the soil being less productive than God intended it to be.

Their disobedience meant physical exertion for Adam and his progeny as they sweated to master the soil. It also meant expulsion from the beautiful Garden of Eden, so that the two of them could not eat of the fruit of the Tree of Life and live forever (Genesis 3:22–24). One can only imagine the sorrow they felt as they left that beautiful place.

Even though sin and death came into the world, the pre-flood period, it is generally believed, was still superior to this present world. It appears that the oceans were smaller in area, since much of the water was in the firmament above the earth, a condition which would have made for healthy living. Fertility of the soil was greater, and the climate was mild and pleasant all over the earth. Both animals and plants, as well as mankind, were larger, healthier, and lived longer than succeeding generations. The food was more nutritious and supplied the needs of all living beings.

No Zero Population

We know that a population explosion took place upon the earth, because the Bible clearly states that this happened (Genesis 6). There were ten generations from Adam to Noah, and if the average family numbered twenty children (a conservative estimate), it is altogether likely that there may have been two billion people or more in the world at the time of the flood.

You Have to Eat

Only one man was a pleasure to the Lord. His name, of course, was Noah. Among the instructions which God gave to Noah regarding the ark and how He was going to save Noah, his family, and pairs of every animal, were these words: "Store away in the boat all the food that they [the animals] and you will need" (Genesis 6:21).

It isn't until after the account of the flood that mention is made of meat. When Noah, his wife, and his sons and their wives disembarked from their floating piece of real estate, God gave instructions once again as to their diets for survival. "Every moving thing that liveth shall be meat for you; even as the green herb have I given you all things. But flesh with the life thereof, which is the blood thereof, shall ye not eat" (Genesis 9:3, 4 KJV). Man's food was to be meat (properly prepared), herbs, grain, vegetables, seeds, and fruit.

There is growing evidence today that meat may be contributing to many of mankind's ills. But in its first use as food, the contaminants did not exist, and man was being told that this was complete protein, which we now know is essential for good health. Protein contains nitrogen; carbohydrates and fats do not.

Food Fit for Angels

The Bible traces the growth of the new race, and finally there emerges the exciting story of Abraham, Isaac, Jacob, and Jacob's children (ending with the death of Joseph in Egypt).

In Genesis 18 we find an interesting account of three angels visiting Abraham. The old patriarch immediately instructed his wife to prepare food for the visitors. It was food fit for angels! There was bread made of three measures of fine meal, tender veal, butter and milk (Genesis 18: 6–8).

Later in the Genesis account, Lot entertains two angels and sets before them a great feast, which included freshly baked unleavened bread (Genesis 19:3).

Anything for Food

A glaring revelation of what man will do for food is dramatically brought out in the story of Esau selling his birthright for a mess of pottage (Genesis 25:29–34). The phrase, "Boy, am I starved!" must have originated with Esau, the skillful hunter.

Isaac's fondness for food was not diminished in his old age. Half-blind and approaching death, he called for Esau, his older son, and instructed him to take his bow and arrow and get him some venison. ". . . prepare it just the way I like it—" he instructed, adding, "savory and good—and bring it here for me to eat . . ." (Genesis 27:2–4).

Rebekah, Isaac's wife, appears on the scene, and overhearing the conversation calls their son Jacob, sharing with him the request of the old gentleman. It is a familiar story—Jacob, carrying out his mother's instructions, gets two young goats which Rebekah fixes and Jacob serves to his father. He was able to accomplish this deceitful act by a clever disguise, and Isaac, his senses dimmed by old age, falls victim to the ruse and gives Jacob his special blessings. The point is, of course, that once again food enters into the transaction.

Food for Survival

There came a turning point in Jacob's life where he wrestled with an angel of the Lord and emerged a changed man. His name was changed to Israel and he became the father of the twelve tribes of Israel. All this is significant as we trace the biblical references to food.

Jacob's sons turned on their brother Joseph and sold him into slavery. Years later, they came face-to-face with the brother they left for dead, when they were forced to go to Egypt in search of grain. A great drought swept across the land. Crop failures and famine were the result; only Egypt had grain. Jacob instructed his sons, "Go down and buy some for us before we all starve to death" (Genesis 42:2).

Joseph was occupying a high place in the affairs of the government of Egypt. In the great, good providence of God, Joseph was able to help his family in this, their dire time of need. The providential significance of this historical situation should not be lost to our thinking. In a highly emotional confrontation, Joseph reveals his identity to his brothers and says, "God has sent me here to keep you and your families alive, so that you will become a great nation" (Genesis 45:7).

As we trace the influence of food, and the need for it for survival, we see the overruling hand of Almighty God in the lives of these who figured so prominently in this period of history.

While in Egypt, the Israelites ate well, according to their own statement. As they wandered in the wilderness (led by Moses and Aaron), they moaned and complained, "Oh, that we were back in Egypt . . . . For there we had plenty to eat. But now you have brought us into this wilderness to kill us with starvation" (Exodus 16:3).

That wasn't true, however, for God gave them a balanced diet and literally rained down food from heaven in the form of meat to eat in the evening, and bread in the morning (vv. 4–9). ". . . the food became known as 'manna' (meaning 'What is it?') . . ." (v. 31). The manna was a carbohydrate, and the quail was the protein their bodies needed.

Once they arrived in the Promised Land, Canaan, they found:

> . . . a good land, a land of brooks of water, of fountains and depths that spring out of the valleys and hills; A land of wheat, and barley, and vines, and fig trees, and pomegranates; a land of oil olive, and honey; A land wherein thou shalt eat bread without scarceness, thou shalt not lack any thing in it . . . .
>   Deuteronomy 8:7–9 KJV

The rules and regulations governing the use of food were given here by God.

2

The Bible, Food, and You

He gives food to every living thing, for his loving-
kindness continues forever.

Psalms 136:25

In this chapter we will consider the foods we find mentioned in the Bible.

Milk and Milk Products

Milk and milk products have always been more generally
used as food by the peoples of the Near East than by ourselves. Not only was the milk of cows used, but that of sheep,
camels, goats, donkeys, and other animals. It is interesting to
note that the Scriptures equate milk, along with honey, as a
symbol of prosperity, describing a goodly land as "flowing
with milk and honey" (Exodus 3:8; Deuteronomy 6:3; 11:9).

Milk was used fresh, but was also used when sour or curdled. (This is not surprising when you consider that there was
no refrigeration.)

Ancient records point to the widespread use of milk. The
walls of tombs show pastoral scenes of cows and their calves.
As far back as 116 to 27 B.C., Roman writers were pointing out
the importance of milk as a food. It is also a matter of record
that when early Christians were baptized they were given
milk and honey to symbolize this important event in their
spiritual lives. From the very beginning of civilization milk
was necessary for survival. It is often called the perfect food.
Nutritionally it provides protein, minerals (in particular calcium and phosphorus), vitamins, and easily digested fat. No
wonder it is the food for infants.

Butter.   Butter is not always called *butter* in the Bible. Sometimes it is called *curds.* The curds could refer to cheese or yogurt as well. But there is ample reference to butter and its use in Bible times. And the butter that is mentioned is no doubt the kind of butter we know today, for in Psalms 55:21 KJV the writer says: "The words of his mouth were smoother than butter . . . ." The Book of Judges tells of butter being served ". . . in a lordly dish" (Judges 5:25 KJV).

Cheese.   The milk product cheese is mentioned specifically in the Bible three times (1 Samuel 17:18; 2 Samuel 17:29; Job 10:10). Job's complaint is graphic: "Hast thou not poured me out as milk, and curdled me like cheese?" (KJV). Actually cottage cheese is the first stage in the cheese-making process, and the comparison no doubt refers to this form of cheese. Cheese is an excellent and inexpensive substitute for meat. This may explain its widespread use by early civilizations. Without refrigeration processes, it would have been very difficult to keep meat from spoiling; therefore cheese was the natural substitute.

Yogurt.   Another milk-product food of ancient origin is yogurt. Sometimes in the Bible it is referred to as *curds.* Yogurt has been called "the food of long life." Americans have been slow to discover yogurt compared to the people in Turkey, Lapland, Iceland, and China, who have been eating it for centuries. One of the most valuable contributions that yogurt makes to one's diet is that it promotes the growth of desirable intestinal bacteria. Not only does yogurt have therapeutic qualities, but its satiny texture is delightful and the flavor unequaled. It is believed that David and his followers were given yogurt with honey to help satisfy their hunger and thirst (2 Samuel 17:29).

Meat and Protein Foods

The eating of the meat of domestic animals came to be strictly regulated by Mosaic Law. There was a large class of animals which was looked upon as ceremonially unfit to be eaten. Leviticus 11 and Deuteronomy 14 spell these prohibitions out in detail. Twenty birds are listed as being unclean and unfit for human consumption (Leviticus 11:13–19). A list of forbidden small animals which scurry about one's feet or crawl upon the ground was also given (Leviticus 11:29, 30).

The kinds of animal food most frequently referred to in the Bible are cattle, sheep, lamb, goat, and various species of wild game, especially the antelope. Lamb is a traditional Easter meat for many Christians, and Jewish custom dictates that it be served at the observance of Passover. Instructions for its preparation are given in Exodus 12:8. Undoubtedly lamb played an important role in the diet of biblical people.

Wild Game.   Animals of field and woods commonly provided food. There are references to Nimrod who was ". . . a mighty hunter before the Lord . . ." (Genesis 10:9 KJV); to Ishmael as the lad who became an archer (Genesis 21:20); and to Esau as the ". . . skillful hunter . . ." (Genesis 25:27).

Fish.   If you were asked to name the food you associate most often with people who lived in Bible times, undoubtedly most readers would say, "Fish." What picture comes to mind as you think of Jesus eating with His disciples? Is it not the scene at the Sea of Galilee when the multitude followed Him? Jesus' concern for their physical well-being is shown as He questions His disciples as to how they were going to feed that immense crowd. Andrew supplies the answer as he tells Jesus of the small lad with five barley loaves and a couple of fish. The story is related in all four Gospels (Matthew 14; Mark 6; Luke 9; John 6). It is an incredible miracle—this feeding of five thousand and then the gathering up afterwards of twelve basketsful of fragments. There is a teaching here that is often overlooked. Jesus cautioned against wastefulness: "Now gather the scraps . . . so that nothing is wasted" (John 6:12).

The Sea of Galilee furnished great quantities of fresh fish. The Israelites had learned in Egypt to highly prize fish as food, and their laws allowed the free use of any fish that had fins and scales (Leviticus 11:9, 10).

One of the first things Jesus did after His Resurrection was to eat a piece of broiled fish, and a honeycomb (Luke 24:42 KJV). Another post-Resurrection account tells of Jesus fixing fish for His disciples on the seashore. It is one of the last things Jesus apparently did for His beloved disciples as recorded by the Apostle John (John 21).

Eggs. Here was another addition to the diet of the Hebrews. Job asks, "Can that which is unsavoury be eaten without salt? or is there any taste in the white of an egg?" (Job 6:6 KJV). Jesus, in teaching about the importance of prayer, referred to several foods, among them eggs (Luke 11:12).

Vegetables and Fruits

The importance of fruit in the diet of early man has been pointed out earlier. Among fruits, the most commonly mentioned is the grape. Noah was a farmer, more specifically, a husbandman who had a vineyard. The grapes in those days must have been of exceptionally large size. One such cluster brought by the spies to Joshua was so large that it required two men to carry it on a pole between them! This same passage tells of the samples of pomegranates and figs which these men brought back (Numbers 13:23).

Grapes then, as today, were eaten fresh, or dried and eaten in the form of raisins. They were also pressed into cakes. But much of the grape crop was made into juice and wine, and also vinegar (Numbers 6:1–4; Ruth 2:14; Matthew 27:34 KJV). The Bible contains warnings against the too-free use of wine and strong drink (Proverbs 20:1; Proverbs 23:29–35; Isaiah 5:22; Isaiah 56:11, 12). The early Christians were told not to eat or drink wine or do anything that would offend a brother or make him sin (Romans 14:21).

Next to the grape, the fig holds the most prominent place among the fruits cultivated by the Israelites. The first fruit to be mentioned by name is the fig (Genesis 3:7). Isaiah prescribed figs to heal King Hezekiah's boils (Isaiah 38:21). Figs were eaten both fresh and in a dried state. When dried they were pressed into a form of round cakes. Figs were thought to have curative properties (2 Kings 20:7). When David and his six hundred men were out after the Amalekites, they found an Egyptian youth who had neither eaten nor drunk anything for three days and nights. What did they give him to eat? Figs, raisins, and water (1 Samuel 30:11, 12).

There are any number of very interesting accounts in the Bible that refer to food being brought as gifts, in some instances as appeasement, at other times as rewards, and still other stories just relating the eating habits of the people. Figs figure very prominently in such accounts (1 Samuel 25:18; Nehemiah 13:15). God, in speaking through the prophet Hosea, speaks of figs as being "satisfying," especially ". . . the early figs of summer in their first season!" (Hosea 9:10). One of the most astonishing events in Jesus' life relates to His reaction to a barren fig tree.

Another fruit that was widely cultivated was the date palm. Dates were eaten fresh or dried. King Solomon's temple was decorated with carvings of the date palm (1 Kings 6:29–32). Jericho is referred to in 2 Chronicles 28:15 as ". . . the City of Palm Trees."

When the Israelites were bitterly complaining on their wilderness trek, one of the things they reminisced about was the fertile land and the wonderful crops they'd left behind, which included figs, vines, and pomegranates (Numbers 20:5).

Another fruit mentioned is the apple (but it may also mean the apricot or quince). Joel laments that "the apples shrivel on the trees . . ." (Joel 1:12).

Vegetables in great variety are mentioned, not only as cultivated products, but as growing wild in the fields. A very interesting story of Naboth's denial of his vineyard to King Ahab is given in 1 Kings 21. The King wanted it for a garden of herbs. Naboth's reply shows the value a man placed on his garden land: "Not on your life! That land has been in my family for generations" (1 Kings 21:3).

Still another incident involved Elisha the prophet (2 Kings 4: 40, 41).

There are references to beans, lentils, cucumbers, melons,

leeks, onions, and even garlic (Genesis 25:34; Numbers 11:5; 2 Samuel 17:28; Isaiah 1:8). Vegetables which now grow in Palestine and likely grew in Bible times are the beet, turnip, radish, carrot, cabbage, eggplant, tomato, and squash.

Condiments, Nuts, Oils, and Sweets

Among *condiments* mentioned in the Bible are mint, anise, dill, cummin, salt, coriander seed, rue, and mustard (Exodus 16:31; Job 6:6; Isaiah 28:27; Matthew 13:31). The value of these things was counted such that the Scribes and Pharisees even used them to pay tithes (Matthew 23:23). Dandelion greens and endive were two of the "bitter herbs" called for in the Passover meal (Exodus 12:8; Numbers 9:11).

Of all the spices mentioned in the Bible, one of the most familiar is the tiny mustard seed and its related parable (Matthew 13:31; Mark 4:31, 32). The other condiment that recalls a biblical illustration has to do with salt and Jesus' reminder to the disciples that we are to be "the salt of the earth" (Matthew 5:13; Mark 9:50 KJV).

There are a few species of *nuts* mentioned in the Bible. When Jacob sent his sons to Egypt for corn (grain), he bade them take with them a present, ". . . a little balm, and a little honey, spices, and myrrh, nuts, and almonds . . ." (Genesis 43:11 KJV). The Book of Ecclesiastes talks of the almond tree flourishing (Ecclesiastes 12:5). And imagine the surprise of the Israelites when Aaron's rod ". . . budded, and brought forth buds, and bloomed blossoms, and yielded almonds" (Numbers 17:8 KJV).

Every serious student of the Bible recognizes the importance of *oil* to the ancient people. Oil was usually pressed from the olive, but also came from roses, nuts, and the castor bean. If you were raised on Bible stories as a child, then you recall the thrill you felt as you heard the story of Elijah and the widow with her meager supply of cooking oil (1 Kings 17:13–16).

The important place in our diet of *sweetening* was supplied in ancient Palestine by honey. It was used to dress up the flavor of other foods, and was itself eaten as a food. We have already made several references to honey and the honeycomb. The ancients apparently knew better than we do of the danger of eating too freely of honey. In Proverbs 25:16 KJV we read, "Hast thou found honey? eat so much as is sufficient for thee, lest thou be filled therewith, and vomit it."

If only we would take to heart these admonitions regarding the consumption of sugar. This is an abuse perpetrated by modern man that has contributed to more of our ills and physical problems than one can possibly imagine. It is believed that sugar is a major contributor to coronary disease. We are, sadly, a sugar-oriented nation, and the results are tragically evident. If we are going to eat our way to good health, then our sugar consumption has got to be drastically reduced.

The natural sweeteners which God placed upon this earth are honey, syrups (from trees), carob powders, and ground dried fruits. Sugar as we know it is not mentioned in the Bible. That is an omission which we need seriously consider as being for our benefit. But of all the biblical foods, honey would have to rank as one of the best loved. The Psalmist refers to it (again as a comparison): "How sweet are thy words unto my taste! yea, sweeter than honey to my mouth!" (Psalms 119:103 KJV).

Breads and Cereals

And what shall one say with regard to breads and cereals and their mention and use in the Bible! The use of a concordance is recommended as you search out the value of breads and cereals as spelled out so clearly. For example, Ezekiel 4:9 shows how the Bible cooks prepared certain kinds of bread. There we are told: ". . . eat bread made of flour mixed from wheat, barley, beans, lentils, and spelt. Mix the various kinds of flour together in a jar."

Bread always constituted a main part of the diet. Properly baked bread, made from the right materials (whole grain flours), has been the staff of life from earliest history, and has always been one of the principal foods that God gave to man.

But it has indeed been made the staff of death by modern milling processes.

We find mention of barley in the Bible. Bible students will quickly recall that when Ruth gleaned in the fields of Boaz, it was barley that she gathered (Ruth 2:17). Remember also that Jesus fed the multitude with barley loaves and fish (John 6:8–13). There are some thirty-two biblical references to this important grain, which formed such a vital part of Bible-time diets.

God-Given Food Rules

Recognition is slowly coming to our civilized world that we are made of the food that we consume and that sickness and disease are largely the result of an improper diet. This overview of some highlights of what the Bible has to say about food is given as a background to help the reader understand that God has clearly set forth the rules that are to govern our eating habits.

In Isaiah 55:2 the prophet wrote: "Why spend your money on foodstuffs that don't give you strength? Why pay for groceries that don't do you any good?" Such biblical guidelines are given for our best interests. Just as in our spiritual lives we deny ourselves the help and hope we so often need, so in our physical bodies we are deprived by a failure to heed the Word of God. It is time that we heed the warnings of nutritionists and others (many of whom have been trying to get the attention of the food-buying public for long years), and that we take seriously all that the Bible has to say about food and the care of our bodies.

3

Fight Self-Pollution

... thou hast withholden bread from the hungry.

Job 22:7 KJV

Are Americans healthy and well-fed? Are you as healthy and well-nourished as you feel you could be? When you look at yourself in the mirror, are you satisfied with the image? Are there telltale signs indicating that you've been putting the wrong things into your mouth? Don't you feel quite up to par? And what of your precious family members?

A travel-magazine article by Robert D. Kilpatrick, president of Connecticut General Life Insurance Company, arrests our attention with its title: "Rising Health-Care Costs—A Drag on the Economy." Health-care costs are a growing concern to business management, because health insurance is a major item in the budget of most businesses. But what of the unfortunate people who have to provide their own insurance! Kilpatrick states that Americans now spend more than $120 billion annually on health, compared to $39 billion a decade ago. Health-care expenditures amount to more than 8 percent of the gross national product, an increase of more than one-third from the 6-percent level of ten years ago. Does it come as a shock to you to learn that, according to one source, the cost of the average hospital stay has increased from $311 in 1965 to more than $1,000 in 1977?

Who Is to Blame?

We are individually responsible for our health and that of our family members. Blame must also be laid at the feet of the Food and Drug Administration, along with the food and beverage industries, and our drug industries. None has been very

23

cautious or strict in enforcement of existing rules and regulations governing the testing, marketing and administration of foods and drugs.

The money spent on drug bills each year amounts to a staggering sum in many households. Reliable sources inform us that half of such drugs are either not needed or are incorrectly prescribed. Prescription drugs are responsible for over 100,000 unnecessary deaths a year, and it is estimated that 30 to 40 percent of all hospital patients suffer adverse drug reactions.

It is encouraging to pick up a major city newspaper and see a headline screaming out: AMERICANS TURNING OUT TO FIGHT HEALTH HAZARDS. The article by William G. Crook, M.D., appeared in *The Houston Post* in the doctor's column, *Child Care.*

A Heaping Serving of a Portion of Death

I wonder how many people who misuse and abuse their bodies stop to realize that they are serving themselves a portion of death. While it is true that today a greater number of Americans survive infancy and childhood diseases, it is a sobering fact that after middle age, men (in particular) are not as healthy as were their grandfathers. It has been said that in this country we have more degenerative diseases than any other people in the world. We're not a healthy nation, and we'd better hasten to face up to the stark reality of that fact.

How many people do you know who are starving for calories? Glance over any group of people and you have to come to the conclusion that the majority of individuals are overstuffed. Notice we did not say well-fed! Many individual diets are lacking in valuable protein, vitamins, minerals, and other nutrients that will insure good health and longevity.

High-risk age groups, which feel the effects of unhealthy eating the most, are infants, small children, teenagers, pregnant and nursing mothers, and the aged. For instance, if their diet during the first two years of life is inadequate nutritionally, children may not develop normally, neither physically nor mentally. A scary thought. Far too many infants in this country are deprived of the one food nature provided for them in such a beautiful way—mother's milk.

Even teenagers from high-income families may be undernourished. In spite of all our abundance, the diet of many young people from affluent homes is incredibly lacking in many of the vital body-building nutrients so essential to physical and mental good health. Teenagers often do not get enough protein to build sound tissues, enough calcium to build strong bones and good teeth, enough B-complex vitamins for steady nerves, enough vitamin A for efficient vision, or enough iron for normal blood. Surveys prove this. One statewide survey showed that only 21 percent of teenage boys and 12 percent of the girls were getting the recommended daily food allowances. Another survey has shown that about one-half of the school children in the United States do not get enough vitamin C, and often show inflammation of the gums and easy bruising.

Older people, many of whom live alone, often do not have an adequate diet. A survey made of 296 elderly people living in two government housing projects showed the following figures:

	Milk	Meat	Vegetables Fruits	Breads Cereals
Inadequate	236	101	148	72
Adequate	60	195	148	224

Many of these elderly people were using no milk at all, which means they would be low in calcium. Those inadequate in the meat group would be low in protein, iron, and some of the B-complex vitamins. Those inadequate in the vegetable and fruit group would be low in vitamins A and C, and in some of the trace minerals. Only a few were inadequate in the bread and cereal group, because when living alone it is easier to make a sandwich or fill up on sweet rolls, toast, and cookies than to prepare a well-balanced meal. Much of the illness of older people is due to poor nutrition rather than old age.

It is an accepted fact that extreme dietary deficiencies can produce diseases such as beriberi, scurvy, xerophthalmia, and pellagra; but it is not generally recognized that lesser deficiencies will produce milder cases of the same condition. An individual can have poor eyesight, be tired or anemic, have bleeding gums, and pains in the joints, without realizing that these are due to nutritional deficiencies.

A Shocking Report

In 1967 Congress directed the Department of Health, Education, and Welfare to determine the scope and location of malnutrition and related health problems in the United States. Research was conducted in ten states and New York City. The clinical evaluation included a medical history, physical examination, anthropometric measurements, X-ray examination of the wrist, dental examination, and hemoglobin and hematocrit determinations. This evaluation involved approximately 40,000 individuals.

Results indicated that a significant proportion of the population surveyed was malnourished or was at a high risk of developing nutritional problems. Findings were reported in *Food and Nutrition,* February 1973:

1. There was increasing evidence of malnutrition as the income level decreased.
2. Adolescents between the ages of ten and sixteen years had the highest prevalence of unsatisfactory nutritional status.
3. Male adolescents had more evidence of malnutrition than females.
4. Persons over sixty showed evidence of gradual undernutrition which was not restricted to the very poor.
5. As the homemaker's educational level increased, the evidence of nutritional inadequacies in the children decreased.
6. Among adults there was also a positive relationship between the number of years of school completed by the individual and his or her nutritional status.
7. Many persons made poor food choices that led to inadequate diets, and to poor use of the money available for food.

8. Many households seldom used foods rich in vitamin A.
9. Many diets were deficient in iron content.
10. In children and adolescents it was found that between-meal snacks of foods high in carbohydrates, such as candies, soft drinks, and pastries were associated with the development of dental cavities.
11. School lunches contributed to a substantial proportion of the total nutrient intake of many school children.
12. Obesity is a nutritionally related problem because of its association with increased rates of diabetes, certain cardiovascular diseases, and other chronic diseases.
13. Iron deficiency anemia, as evidenced by a high prevalence of low levels of hemoglobin, is a widespread problem and is due largely to nutritional iron deficiency.
14. A relatively large proportion of pregnant and lactating women demonstrated low serum-albumin levels, suggesting marginal protein nutrition in this group.
15. Young people in all groups had a high prevalence of low vitamin A levels.
16. Males generally had a higher prevalence of low vitamin C levels than did females. The prevalence of poor vitamin C status increased with age.
17. Riboflavin status was poor among blacks and among young people of all groups.

What can we do about this situation? First of all, as Christians, we must realize that all creation is in bondage to sin:

For all creation is waiting patiently and hopefully for that future day when God will resurrect his children. For on that day thorns and thistles, sin, death, and decay—the things that overcame the world against its will at God's command—will all disappear, and the world around us will share in the glorious freedom from sin which God's children enjoy. For we know that even the things of nature, like animals and plants, suffer in sickness and death as they await this great event. And even we Christians, although we have the Holy Spirit within us as a foretaste of future glory, also groan to be released from

pain and suffering. We, too, wait anxiously for that day when
God will give us our full rights as his children, including the
new bodies he has promised us—bodies that will never be sick
again and will never die.

Romans 8:19–23

What conclusion can be reached? Much of society has ig-
nored for too long the implications of what a wrong diet does
to one's health. When you read a medical bulletin stating that
80 percent of the cancer cases in this country are the result of
pollution, then you should sit up and take notice. This pollution affects our food, not just our environment. We *are* what
we eat. Our mental and emotional stability, or lack of it, is
directly traceable to the foods we consume. Our total physical
well-being is dependent on nourishing every vital organ. It's
time for you to join in the fight against self-pollution.

4

The Basic Four

For the earth has yielded abundant harvests.
Psalms 67:6

The Basic Four is a simple device for planning adequate nutrition on a daily basis. It allows for a variety of foods that will provide a well-balanced diet that includes essential nutrients. The food groups mentioned in this Basic Four plan are: (1) milk and its products; (2) meats, poultry, fish, eggs, and other excellent protein sources; (3) vegetables and fruits; and (4) cereals and their products. We have already considered what the Bible has to say about the different food groups, but specific observations are in order as to present-day usage of the Basic Four.

The Milk Group

The milk group includes all forms of liquid milk, cheese, ice cream, and other milk-based foods. Children should have three or more glasses of milk daily, teenagers and pregnant and nursing mothers four or more glasses, and adults two or more glasses. This does not all have to be taken as liquid milk, but part of it can be from cheese, ice cream, custard, creamed soups, and so on.

Milk is very essential in the diet, as it is our best food source of calcium. It is also a good source of protein and of riboflavin—a B-complex vitamin.

But what if milk cannot be taken, due to an allergy, lack of the enzyme lactase, or a violent dislike for milk? Since calcium is a nutrient that would be lacking if milk were not consumed, it is possible to substitute bonemeal tablets, calcium lactate or calcium gluconate tablets, or dolomite tablets. Foods from the meat group could be increased to provide the protein lacking when milk is not used.

Fluid milk may be whole or skim, buttermilk, evaporated milk, or in powdered form. If cheese or ice cream replaces part of the milk, the portions of their milk equivalents in calcium are:

1-inch cube of cheddar cheese = ½ cup milk
½ cup cottage cheese = ⅓ cup milk
2 tablespoons cream cheese = 1 tablespoon milk
½ cup ice cream = ¼ cup milk

What about using butter? There are those who question the wisdom of using butter, believing that it contributes to cholesterol problems. Adelle Davis discovered in her research that butterfat appears to be a problem only when nutrients needed to utilize it are undersupplied. (See her book *Let's Get Well*.) Miss Davis was always cautious about using margarines. She recommended that a modified butter be prepared by allowing a pound of butter to warm to room temperature and blending it with a liquefier made of one cup of pressed soy, safflower, or peanut oil, and then molding it in an ice tray. The flavor is excellent, and the fatty acids necessary for the body are readily provided.

Fats as such are not mentioned in the Basic Four food groups, but there are fats in whole milk, cheese, meats, and eggs. The fat in the milk group and meat group provides us with sufficient amounts (and in many instances too much), but this is mostly saturated fat since it is from animal sources. These fats may increase the blood cholesterol and triglycerides.

It is recommended that we have two tablespoons of liquid vegetable oil in some form daily to provide us with certain essential fatty acids which the body must have, and to balance the saturated fats in meat, eggs and milk. The best sources of vegetable fat are safflower oil, corn oil, soybean oil, and cottonseed oil, in that order. It can also be obtained from salad dressings, mayonnaise, nuts, sunflower seeds, avocados, or old-fashioned (unhydrogenated) peanut butter.

Studiously avoid foods labeled *hydrogenated*. In the process of hydrogenation, hydrogen is added to unsaturated fats (the vegetable oils which are by nature liquid) to give them a solid consistency. The advantage for the manufacturer is simple—the products keep well, they cost less, and they bring higher profits. Some hydrogenated end-products are baked goods, non-dairy substitutes, imitation milk, processed peanut butter, and many convenience foods.

Do read labels when purchasing cheese. Search for natural cheeses as opposed to processed cheeses. Many additives are added to cheese products, and even those labeled *natural* may not be as natural as one might suppose. But cheese is an excellent source of protein and contains more essential amino acids than do vegetable proteins.

The Meat-Protein Group

The meat group includes the usual animal foods such as beef, veal, lamb, pork, and venison; and variety meats such as liver, heart and kidney. Also included are poultry and eggs. Fish would be considered part of the "meat group" in the Basic Four. Liver is the most nutritious form of meat available.

It is recommended that two or more servings from the meat group be eaten every day. A serving is three ounces of lean cooked meat, poultry, or fish (boneless). Much is being written warning against using meat and poultry because of unnatural farming methods used in raising animals and poultry. Some individuals claim they feel 100 percent better since cutting back drastically on meat consumption, if not cutting it out altogether.

We know our foods are altered these days; we are a drug-oriented, profit-motivated country, and this is reflected in the food industries as well as other places. The worst offenders are hot dogs, luncheon meats, sausage, bacon, ham, and ground beef.

What is a person to do? We know that animal foods contain complete protein; that is, all of the essential amino acids are present. We know that the human body contains more than

100,000 different kinds of protein. Did you know, for instance, that your hair is 97 percent protein? So protein in some form equal to our daily needs is absolutely essential. The individual reader must decide whether meat will contribute the larger share of protein to his diet, or whether he will search out other forms of protein.

If you are going to eat meat, you must make certain it is well cooked. The warning needs to be sounded in particular if one is going to eat pork, for the danger of trichinosis does exist. Trichinosis is the disease that comes from the trichina worm, which is found in hogs. This is a very real danger that far too many people refuse to admit exists.

Virginia and Norman Rohrer suggest in *How to Eat Right and Feel Great* that soybeans are "tomorrow's meat for a burgeoning world," and further state:

> . . . the grain-cattle-meat cycle robs the world of vegetable protein which, if not fed to cattle, could keep many people alive. Next time you select an eight-ounce steak at the supermarket's meat counter, look around. There are forty-five starving people standing with empty bowls which could have been filled with the grain it took to grow that piece of meat.
>
> Protein derived from animal sources is too expensive for most families in the global community of four billion people. Soon animal protein may be unavailable at any price. Production of meat protein requires a costly double cycle: the crops draw their nourishment from soil, the animals eat the crops and turn it into protein, the animals are then slaughtered and eaten to provide protein that originated with the crops for the diet of man.

The Rohrers' concern is not only for the health of the world's billions, but in survival for a population curve that continues to spiral upward at an alarming rate. They and others are taking up the cry, warning that new sources of protein must be found and tapped if the multiplied billions in tomorrow's world are to be fed adequately. One logical solution may be to turn to soybeans.

If you are going to rule out meat, or are going to cut back on your meat consumption, then you must take steps to make certain you obtain sufficient protein from milk, cheese, eggs, dry beans, peas, and nuts.

The important thing is to get the nutrients that one's body requires. For example, vitamin B_{12} cannot be obtained from plant foods.

The Vegetable and Fruit Group

Four or more servings of vegetables and fruits are recommended every day. A serving is the equivalent of the following:

> ½ cup of vegetable or fruit
> 1 medium apple, banana, orange, or potato
> Half a medium grapefruit or cantaloupe
> The juice of one lemon

Include one serving of a good source of vitamin A; the remaining two or three servings may be of any vegetable or fruit. Vitamin A is associated with deep color, so the dark green and deep yellow vegetables are rich in it. This would include broccoli, carrots, chard, collards, watercress, kale, pumpkin, spinach, sweet potato, and winter squash. Fruits that are good sources of vitamin A would include apricots, cantaloupe, mango, papaya, and persimmon.

Excellent sources of vitamin C are oranges and orange juice, grapefruit or grapefruit juice, cantaloupe, mango, papaya, raw strawberries, broccoli, Brussels sprouts, red and green peppers. Other sources are honeydew melon, lemons, tangerines or tangerine juice, watermelon, asparagus tips, raw cabbage, mustard greens and all other greens, potatoes and sweet potatoes (cooked in their jackets), spinach, and tomatoes or tomato juice.

Of course, vegetables and fruits are great sources of iron and trace minerals such as potassium and magnesium, and the importance of minerals to one's health cannot be overemphasized. Nerve-cell membranes are particularly affected by both a deficiency or an excess of minerals within the body, and there are tests that can be taken to determine your mineral levels.

The roughage to be obtained from vegetables and fruits is also vital for good elimination.

"Mary, Mary . . . how does your garden grow?" This is a good place to suggest that you give thought to growing your own vegetables. Even a small garden plot can furnish enough vegetables for a family of four. A couple of rows of radishes, lettuce, carrots, beets, and so on, with one-half dozen tomato plants and some green beans running up poles or around a fence will furnish all the vegetables a family can eat, and even leave some for freezing. The savings in money, the satisfaction and delight in seeing one's garden produce, and the added benefit of taste, make the venture worth every effort.

Fruits are best when eaten fresh and/or raw. If you have experienced the joys of having fruit trees around your home, then you know that nothing is more delicious than fully ripened, freshly picked fruit. If you are considering planting trees, why not give some consideration to fruit trees? If you have been giving your family "empty-calorie" cake, cookies or other desserts, now is the time to recognize the need for change and start serving fresh fruit instead.

The Bread and Cereal Group

This group includes not only breads, quick breads and other baked goods, but cereals (both ready-to-eat and cooked varieties), cornmeal, crackers, flours, grits, bulgur, macaroni, spaghetti, noodles, rice, and rolled oats. Choose four or more servings daily. Count as one serving the following:

One slice of bread
One ounce of ready-to-eat cereal
½ to ¾ cup of cooked cereal, cornmeal, grits, macaroni, spaghetti, noodles, or rice

In recent years much has been made of the "new" findings that fiber is vital to health. It is really nothing new. The Bible has always proclaimed this! Lack of fiber contributes to a vast variety of diseases especially common to Western-civilized man. Dr. David Reuben and Dr. T. L. Cleave have successfully called attention to the fact that refining carbohydrates and stripping our foods of their natural roughage are major contributing causes of diverticular diseases, cancer of the colon, digestive, circulatory, and other diseases.

The diseases which are so common to our society today were unknown to our ancestors for many thousands of years. The evidence is overwhelmingly clear, and should be sufficient to alert even the most skeptical, but still there are those who will buy and set before their unsuspecting families that soft, white, depleted stuff called "bread." Do not be deceived into thinking that, by buying something that says "enriched," you are getting what you need. In his book *Enriched Food—Less Nutrition at Higher Cost,* Ray Wolfe states that "the only things that become enriched are the pockets of the manufacturers."

In the refining process, the milling removes the following percentages of essential elements and minerals:

76% of the iron	86% of the manganese
71% of the phosphorus	89% of the cobalt
77% of the potassium	68% of the copper
85% of the magnesium	78% of the zinc
78% of the sodium	48% of the molybdenum
40% of the chromium	

The answer is to be found in eating breads, cookies, muffins, and other foods of this nature that contain only whole-grain flours. Today's wise homemaker will learn the art of substitution, i.e., substituting nutritious and flavorful whole-grain flours for white flours. This is not a difficult practice, and in your baking you can master it by doing the following: Instead of 1 cup white flour, substitute ¾ cup whole-grain flour; use 1 tablespoon less oil and add 1 to 2 tablespoons more liquid.

You will find that your baking produces cakes, muffins, cookies, and breads that are coarser, but you will also make the grand discovery that they are far more satisfying to the palate. Keep your whole-grain flour in the refrigerator, since it easily becomes infested with weevils.

When it comes to eating cereals, exercise the same precautions as in your choice of breads and related products. Natural whole-grain varieties, which do not contain chemical additives, sugar, or honey, should be your choice. Try making your own granola (see recipe section).

Foods Not in the Four Food Groups

Sugar is not included in this daily food guide, yet sugar *is* found in baked goods, canned fruit, sugar-coated cereals, jams, jellies, soft drinks, and other foods. Sugar has no protein, vitamins, or minerals, and when eaten in large quantities replaces the good foods which do provide those things.

Up to two hundred years ago, refined sugar was unknown. Sweetening agents were honey, maple syrup, sorghum, and molasses. Each person ate between ten and fifteen pounds of those natural sweeteners a year. Today the consumption of sugar varies from about 104 to 170 pounds per person a year in this country. This is all "empty" calories, replacing the good foods of the four food groups. The average person consumes about 500 calories daily in sugar and sweets.

Dr. John Yudkin, an English nutritionist, in his book *Sweet and Dangerous*, attributes heart attacks and other disorders to an excessive use of sugar. He says that sugar is the culprit, rather than fatty foods, in causing atherosclerosis and heart attacks. He tells of the Yemenites who migrated to Israel and whose incidence of heart attacks began to rise at once. Heart attacks were rare on their previous diet, which was moderate in fats but low in sugar. It was a diet very similar to that of the people of Bible days; now refined sugar is available everywhere in Israel.

This same doctor found, in experiments with rats, that a

high sugar diet raises both cholesterol and triglycerides in their blood. Other conditions associated with high sugar consumption are diabetes, excessive stomach acidity, myopia, tooth decay, gout, and obesity.

Hidden Sugars in Common Foods. You may think you are not eating much sugar if, for instance, you do not put sugar in your coffee. But what about the hidden sugars? The columns below give you some idea as to the amount of sugar you may be consuming albeit unknowingly (adapted from *Diet and Dental Health,* American Dental Association, 1963, and current publications on food values.

Food	Serving	Teaspoons of Sugar
Candies (from 75 to 85% sugar)		
Chocolate bar	average size	7
Chocolate mints	1 medium (20/lb.)	3
Cracker Jack, Fiddle Faddle or Zonkers	2 cups	4½
Licorice	long rope	6
Lifesavers	1	⅓
Marshmallow	1 average (60/lb.)	1½
Cake		
Angel food	2¾″ wedge	8
Coffee cake	1 average piece	4½
Cheesecake	4 oz.	7
Chocolate (iced)	1/12 of cake	15
Cupcake (iced)	2″	6
Doughnut (plain)	1	4
Pineapple upside-down	3″ square	15
Cookies		
Brownies, no icing	2″ x 2″ x ¾″	4
Chocolate chip	1	2
Oatmeal	1	1½
Oreo	1	1½

Food	Serving	Teaspoons of Sugar
Custard, Gelatin		
Brown Betty	½ cup	9
Custard, baked	½ cup	4
Fruit-flavored gelatin	½ cup	4–6
Frozen Desserts		
Ice cream	⅛ quart	5–6
Ice cream cone	cone only	3½
Sherbet	⅛ quart	6–8
Pie		
Apple	⅙ (9″ pie)	8
Banana cream	⅙ (9″ pie)	5–6
Cherry or berry	⅙ (9″ pie)	10–11
Custard, coconut	⅙ (9″ pie)	6
Lemon	⅙ (9″ pie)	13–14
Pecan	⅙ (9″ pie)	13
Pumpkin (no whipped cream)	⅙ (9″ pie)	8
Spreads		
Frosting	1 ounce	5
Honey	1 Tbsp.	3
Jam, jelly	1 Tbsp.	3
Maple syrup	1 Tbsp.	2½
Milk Drinks		
Chocolate	1 cup (5 oz. milk)	6
Instant Breakfast	8 ounces (made with milk, chocolate flavor)	2
Milk shake	10 ounces	5
Soft Drinks		
Ginger ale	6 ounces	3⅓
Lemonade	8 ounces	8
Koolaid	8 ounces	6
Carbonated beverage	6 ounces	3 ⅓–4⅓

Food	Serving	Teaspoons of Sugar
Cooked Fruits		
Applesauce (sweetened)	½ cup (scant)	5
Fruit cocktail	½ cup (scant)	5
Peaches, canned in syrup	2 halves, 1 Tbsp. juice	3½
Prunes, stewed (sweetened)	4–5 med., 2 Tbsp. juice	8
Dried Fruits		
Apricots	4–6 halves	4
Dates	3–4	4½
Prunes	3–4 medium	4
Raisins	¼ cup	4
Miscellaneous		
Catsup	2 Tbsp.	1½
Cereal, sugar coated	¾ cup	3–6
Pop Tart (and similar)	1 tart	4½–6

Salt and Other Condiments.   Most people consume too much salt. Salt is thought to be one factor in bringing about high blood pressure, as the incidence of high blood pressure parallels salt intake. The use of iodized salt is recommended to prevent goiter.

Herbs.   There is a growing interest in herbs today, both for eating purposes and for medicinal reasons. Modern medical science is beginning to confirm what the Bible has said from the time of Creation. Dr. Paavo Airola, in *How to Get Well*, says: ". . . man's best medicine is right close to him and all around him—in the plant kingdom. There is not a single disease in man that does not have a corresponding remedy or cure in some herb, root, bark or other botanical medicine. As it is said, 'for every disease there is a cure,' and this cure was given to man by a wise and loving Creator right in his close environment—in the plant kingdom. It behooves us to learn about and use these God-given herbal remedies to cure our ills." Dr. Airola recommends that families try growing herbs in their own yards and/or looking around their own environment for those that may be growing wild.

Herbs are not only valuable for botanical medicines. More and more people are discovering the taste thrills of herbs and what they can do to make meals more enjoyable and inviting. Herb gardens on windowsills have become big business. Some of the most unusual and satisfying beverages can be made from various herbs. Herb teas are increasingly popular, and are known to have mildly calming effects. Gourmet cooks have long known what the addition of herbs does for a recipe.

Beverages. These are not listed in the food groups, except for milk and juices. The most common nonalcoholic beverages consumed in this country are coffee, tea, and cola-carbonated drinks. Research has recently been done on the effects of their caffeine content on the human body. Coffee contains 100 to 150 mgs. of caffeine per cup, tea about 90 mgs., a 12-ounce bottle of a cola drink about 40 to 72 mgs., and a cup of cocoa about 50 mgs.

According to one pediatrician, cola drinks are a cause of insomnia and hyperactivity among children. The medical profession acknowledges that caffeine is addictive. Addiction to caffeine is most prevalent in waitresses, long-distance truck drivers, night-shift workers, and people who drink as many as fifteen to twenty cups of coffee a day.

People who drink more than five cups of coffee a day are more subject to heart attacks than people who drink less coffee. The Harvard School of Public Health found that heavy coffee drinkers were also more susceptible to cancer of the bladder. A German study indicated that in higher organisms caffeine may cause mutations. Some experiments indicate that even the small amount of caffeine present in a cup or two of coffee a day might cause birth defects, and it is suggested that pregnant women reduce or totally eliminate their consumption of caffeine-containing beverages.

A growing percentage of the people of our nation are victims of hypoglycemia, or low blood sugar. One of the contributing causes is the addiction of so many people to carbonated drinks. The facts are there for anyone who is willing to take the time to be informed. If you (or someone you know) are having difficulty with nervousness, irritability, lethargy, insomnia, headaches, heart palpitations, irregular heartbeats, even nausea, diarrhea, and other disturbing problems—stop and think about how much actual caffeine you may be consuming in the course of a day.

It's time we break some very bad habits and consider our accountability to our Creator. "Your own body does not belong to you," the Bible says. "For God has bought you with a great price." Paul the Apostle makes that statement in 1 Corinthians 6:19, 20. We wonder why we aren't feeling well; we pray for better health, but we persist in our old ways of eating and doing things. We must be grieving the father-heart of God.

5

Foundations of Nutrition

Nutrition is a personal matter, as personal as your
diary or income-tax report . . . . To a considerable
degree, your nutrition can give you a coddled-egg
personality or make you a human dynamo. In short,
it can determine your zest for life, the good you put
into it, and the fulfillment you get from it.

Adelle Davis

Our Cellular Structure

The human body, so wonderfully made, is composed of billions of tiny cells. No one describes how we are made in more
beautiful language than the Psalmist:

You made all the delicate, inner parts of my body, and knit
them together in my mother's womb. Thank you for making
me so wonderfully complex! It is amazing to think about. Your
workmanship is marvelous—and how well I know it. You were
there while I was being formed in utter seclusion! You saw me
before I was born and scheduled each day of my life before I
began to breathe. Every day was recorded in your Book!

Psalms 139:13–16

God has put into the earth all the inorganic minerals and
elements which the human body needs for optimum health.
Plants have the power to take the inorganic minerals out of the
soil and, through the action of sunlight, air, and water, change
them into the organic living form that can be used by us. The
"civilized" diet of refined, chemicalized, demineralized, devitalized, artificially colored, and flavored food bears little resemblance to what God intended it to be!

Richard A. Passwater, in his book *Supernutrition,* says that research has forced him to conclude that more than half a million Americans die prematurely each year because of inadequate nutrition. He says that the standard American diet is dangerously deficient in the nutrients essential to good health. As a result, millions of Americans are consigned to years of struggle with debilitating diseases and victimized by fatal ailments that rob them of decades of disease-free life.

Dr. Jean Meyer, of Harvard's Department of Nutrition and chairman of the 1969 White House Conference on Food, Nutrition and Health, reported in *Science* (April 21, 1972): "Malnutrition, whether caused by poverty or improper diet, contributes to the alarming health situation in the United States today . . . . Indeed—in almost thirty nations, life expectancies for adult males have been [since 1950] greater than they were in the United States."

Adelle Davis looked upon the situation in our country as another Fall-of-Rome-type condition. She saw the tremendous increase in ill-health paralleling the ever-mounting consumption of sweets, refined foods, and soft drinks, and the corresponding decreased use of fresh vegetables, whole-grain breads and cereals, legumes and fruits. She maintained that the idea that America was the best-fed nation in the world was propaganda.

We may be the most abundantly fed, she said, but our diets are far from being the best nutritionally. (*See* her *Let's Get Well.*)

What Does the Body Require?

The foods we eat have basically three jobs to perform in our bodies.

First, food provides materials for the body's building and repair. Protein, minerals, and water are what our tissues and bones are made of.

Second, food provides regulators that enable the body to use the materials put into it and to run smoothly. Vitamins are needed for this, and also minerals and protein.

Third, food provides fuel for the body's energy and warmth. Fats and carbohydrates are mainly used for fuel.

A Look at Proteins

Protein is the chief tissue builder. It is the basic substance of every cell in the body. Protein supplies amino acids, which become the building blocks from which body tissue is made. So protein must come first. Twenty-two amino acids commonly occur in proteins. It is from this group that various combinations of amino acids are united to form the proteins occurring in plants and animals. Plants are the original protein source, but milk, cheese, meat, fish, poultry, and eggs are all important in the diet for their abundance of nutritionally complete proteins.

Before these proteins can be used by our cell tissues, they must be changed into different forms. This is the work of enzymes (which act like the worker ants in an anthill), as they break down the molecules and promote digestive chemical reactions.

You Mean I Do Need Fats?

Fats make up part of the structure of cells and form a protective cushion around vital organs and spare protein. They also supply energy, carry the fat-soluble vitamins A, D, E and K, and help the body use them. Fats supply essential fatty acids (found in plant oils such as safflower, corn, cottonseed, soybean, sesame, and wheat germ—all polyunsaturated fats).

Much controversy and confusion has arisen over cholesterol and the supposed need to eliminate eggs and fats from the diet, since they were believed to be the primary contributing causes of heart attacks. Richard Passwater believes this to be a myth. He demonstrates that low-cholesterol diets do not *prevent* heart disease, while high-cholesterol diets do not *cause* heart disease. It is his contention that many Americans are doing themselves far more harm than good by drastically cutting down on their intake of butter, whole milk, and eggs.

The point of bringing all of this to your attention is to urge you to exercise good judgment. Moderation in all things is always to be preferred to an excess of anything. Cholesterol is needed to some extent to help synthesize the bile acids required for digestion and absorption of fats in the intestine, and also to manufacture steroid hormones and vitamin D. If all this sounds complicated, just remember that you don't want to plug and clog your arteries, but if your diet is adequate in all areas and your liver is functioning, it will produce lecithin, which breaks up the cholesterol and moves it along.

The Carbohydrate Culprit

Carbohydrates are the culprit in far too many diets. These are the hidden sweets which stimulate the blood sugar to peak quickly, giving us a lift, but then when insulin is secreted, it causes the sugar level to fall again and the lift doesn't last. Lassitude, fatigue, nervousness, irritability, even exhaustion and foggy thinking are widespread—and why?

Your selection of food at breakfast can prevent or produce fatigue throughout the day. A high-carbohydrate breakfast (orange juice, toast, jelly, a packaged cereal and coffee [both with sugar and milk]) will put sugar into your blood instantly, but it will not last. A breakfast high in protein (eggs, cottage cheese, whole-wheat toast) will get the day's work done and produce a zest for living.

The concentrated carbohydrates found in cane and beet sugars, jellies, jams, candy, and other sweets should be avoided. The natural sugars found in fruits, honey, molasses, and maple syrup should be used in moderation to provide sweetening.

Admittedly, the ideal intake of refined carbohydrates for most individuals would be zero. You might be able to exclude all such carbohydrates (primarily sugar) from your diet for a time, but the hidden sugars will creep back into one's way of eating from time to time. What can be done? An increase of roughage (fiber in the diet) is advisable. This can be done by eating adequate amounts of fruits, vegetables, bran, oatmeal, and whole wheat. One can help to metabolize one's diet through the use of vitamin and mineral supplements.

6

Vitaminizing and Mineralizing
Your Body

But he [God] has always given proof of himself by
the good things he does: he gives you rain from
heaven and crops at the right times; he gives you
food and fills your hearts with happiness.

Acts 14:17 TEV

It is relatively easy for you to secure for yourself and your
family the proper proteins, carbohydrates and fats; but to cap-
ture the vitamins, minerals, trace minerals, and enzymes is a
more difficult feat. These valuable substances, which are absolutely essential to good health, are plentiful in raw vegetables and fruits.

Our muscles, bones, and organs are in the process of con-
tinually being worn and rebuilt. It is obvious that adequate
nutrition is necessary if we are to build better bodies. To gam-
ble with one's health, and the health of family members, is not
only foolish, but we consider it to be in disobedience to the
One who so lovingly fashioned us.

Vim, vigor and vitality can be attained and maintained
through fortifying the body with the vitamins and minerals
that are all-essential. This will bring about a return to good
health, and even slow down or reverse the aging process. You
can be a charming, vivacious, vital young person at seventy; or
a dull, bloated, worn-out, depleted old person at thirty. It all
depends on how alert you are to your needs and how well you
go about taking care of yourself.

Making Old Age Wait

All diseases are caused by chemicals, and all diseases can be cured by chemicals. All the chemicals used by the body— except for the oxygen which we breathe and the water which we drink—are taken in through food. If we only knew enough, all diseases could be prevented, and could be cured, through proper nutrition . . . .

As tissues become damaged, they lack the chemicals of good nutrition, they tend to become old. They lack what we call "tissue integrity." There are people of 40 whose brains and arteries are senile. If we can help the tissues repair themselves by correcting nutritional deficiencies, we can make old age wait.

ADELLE DAVIS
Let's Eat Right to Keep Fit

A View of Vitamins

A man by the name of Casimir Funk first coined the word *vitamine* in 1912 to describe certain food factors which were found to be essential to the maintenance of life. Since then, as more discoveries have been made, researchers have given names to these various complex substances, and we know them today as vitamins A, B_1, B_2, B_6, B_{12}, C, D, E, F, K, L, M, P, Niacin, Biotin, Pantothenic Acid, Folic Acid, Para-amino benzoic acid (or PABA), choline and inositol. There may be other vitamins not yet discovered which will be identified and named in time.

Ideally, all vitamins, minerals, and other nutrients should be obtained from foods. One wishes that it were not necessary to supplement one's diet with vitamins and minerals, but more and more people are feeling the need to do this in order to fill the nutritional gaps produced by nutritionally inferior foods and by our own faulty eating habits.

A book such as this cannot go into great detail regarding the complex role of vitamins and minerals. We will aim to point out specifics regarding these chemical compounds and their primary role in helping regulate your body functions and your personality.

Some Quick *Did You Knows*

Did you know that *without*

Vitamin A—you could not see?
Vitamin B—you could not keep warm?
Vitamin C—you could not stop germ invasion?
Vitamin D—you could not have developed in the first place?
Vitamin E—you could not move a muscle?
Vitamin F—you could not breathe or absorb oxygen?
Vitamin G—you could not think?
Vitamin K—the blood would leak through your blood-vessel walls?

Did you know that vitamins A and C and the minerals calcium and iron are most frequently found short in diets? These are really some elemental facts, but how often when we prepare menus and meals for our families, or when we dine out in restaurants, do we think of these things?

The "Magic" of Minerals

Never underestimate the importance of minerals to your total well-being. Every mineral has a distinct function to perform, which explains why they are called building stones. Minerals that the body requires in large doses are commonly called *macrominerals,* and those needed in smaller doses are called *microminerals,* or *trace minerals.*

Calcium. In combination with phosphorus, calcium is necessary for the formation of strong bones and teeth. Ninety-nine percent of the calcium in our bodies is found in bones and teeth, and one percent in soft tissues and blood. Normal blood contains from 9–11 milligrams of calcium per 100 cubic centimeters. It is essential for the normal clotting of blood, and for normal functioning of nerve tissue. It is also essential for a normal pulse and heart contraction. A magnesium deficiency may lead to a depositing of calcium in soft tissues, and to abnormal bone structure.

If a child gets too little calcium in his food, his bones will be malformed and he may develop rickets. Older people who do not get enough calcium may have brittle bones that break easily and mend slowly. This is the cause of so many slow-to-mend broken hips in the elderly.

The only really good food sources of calcium are milk, milk products such as cheese, and foods made with milk. Other rather small sources of food calcium are shellfish, egg yolk, canned sardines and salmon *with the bones,* soybeans, and green vegetables. Anyone who neglects providing sufficient calcium in the diet pays a heavy price in irritable nerves, decayed teeth, and broken bones.

Iodine. This mineral is very essential, even though only small amounts are needed. It is used by the thyroid gland to form thyroid hormone. If it is deficient, a goiter develops (an enlargement of the thyroid gland). Too little iodine in soil and water is often found in areas away from the seacoast. There is a "goiter belt" across the northern part of the United States. People living there do not get enough iodine. Because of this, iodine is now added to table salt.

Sodium. Most sodium is ingested as sodium chloride, which is ordinary table salt. The normal intake of sodium chloride may range from 2 to 20 grams; 5 grams is a liberal allowance. Most people eat too much salt, and this may lead to high blood pressure and certain heart and kidney conditions. Foods high in salt are processed meats and fish, canned vegetables, and most cheeses. Most fresh vegetables, fruits, and unprocessed cereals contain only a little salt and may be used freely.

Potassium. The dietary need for potassium roughly equals that of sodium. They balance each other. Potassium deficiency can result from protracted diarrhea, diabetic acidosis, and abnormal kidney function. It is manifested by muscular weakness, increased nervous irritability, mental disorientation, and cardiac irregularities. However, dietary deficiency does not exist under ordinary circumstances. When a diuretic is taken over a prolonged time, a potassium deficiency could occur. Caution should be taken in drinking excessive amounts of coffee or tea, as these are diuretics. Fruits, vegetables, and nuts are good sources of potassium, as are unprocessed meats and fish.

Magnesium. Muscle and nerve tissue depend upon a proper balance between calcium and magnesium for normal function. A deficiency of magnesium is manifested by muscle tremor and, in extreme cases, by convulsions. Men daily require about 400 milligrams of magnesium, and women about 300 milligrams, except when pregnant. Then 450 milligrams are required. A normal well-balanced diet of natural foods will provide this amount, but a diet of mostly processed foods will not. Best food sources of magnesium are nuts and whole-grain cereals and breads. Well-known supplements are magnesium oxide and dolomite.

Trace Minerals. There are a number of minerals which are required by man in very small amounts. Copper, cobalt, zinc, manganese, molybdenum, fluorine, selenium, and chromium are all known to be essential, but exact amounts have not been determined.

Iron. As it is used in the formation of red blood cells which carry oxygen from the lungs to each body cell, iron is a very necessary mineral. Too low a consumption of iron-rich food produces anemia. All that talk on TV about "tired blood" is true. Iron is needed for red, healthy blood.

Those persons especially needing larger amounts of iron are babies and young children, teenage girls, women of childbearing age, and pregnant and nursing mothers. The recommended daily allowance for men is only 10 milligrams, but for women it is 18 milligrams. It now appears that most women cannot get enough iron from food sources alone, and should take iron supplements. It is estimated that 60 percent of the body iron is in the blood. Since the life of a blood cell is from three to four months, it is easy to understand why a rich supply of iron is essential, and why it must be constant throughout life.

The daily requirement of the body is actually quite small for some of these minerals, but the regular health demand is persistent and perpetual. If you can visualize your cells as building blocks, and minerals as the ingredients so essential to every block, then you will better understand how necessary it is that we have foods rich in all these essentials. Someone has said, "Good food is the best medicine." Anyone who understands the functions of the cells of the body would agree.

The Leader Nutrients

This chapter can best be concluded by including a chart showing what are called the "Leader Nutrients," the foods that supply these nutrients in important amounts, and the reasons why you need these nutrients from these foods.

Nutrient	Important Food Sources	Use in the Body
Protein	Meat, fish, poultry, eggs Cheese Milk Cereals and breads Dried beans and peas Peanut butter, nuts	To build and repair all tissues in the body To help form substances in the blood which are called "antibodies" and which fight infection To supply energy
Fat	Butter and cream Salad oils and dressings Cooking and table fats Fatty meats	To supply a large amount of energy in a small amount of food To help keep skin smooth and healthy by supplying substances called "essential fatty acids" To carry vitamins A, D, E, K
Carbohydrate (Sugars and Starch)	Breads and cereals Potatoes and corn Dried fruits, sweetened fruits Fresh fruits (smaller amounts) Sugar, syrup, jelly, jam, honey	To supply energy
Vitamin A	Yellow fruits, dark green and deep yellow vegetables Butter, whole milk, vitamin-A-fortified skim milk, cream, cheddar-type cheese, ice cream Liver, eggs	To help keep skin smooth and soft To help keep mucous membranes firm and resistant to infection To protect against night blindness and promote healthy eyes

	Food Sources	Function
B vitamins Thiamin, Riboflavin, and Niacin	Meat, fish, and poultry Eggs, dried peas and beans Milk, cheese, and ice cream Whole grain and enriched breads and cereals White potatoes	To play a central role in the release of energy from food To help the nervous system function properly To help keep appetite and digestion normal
Vitamin B_6	Meats Potatoes, dark green, leafy vegetables Whole grains and dry beans	To help keep skin healthy
Vitamin B_{12}	Milk, cheese Eggs and meats	To help prevent anemia
Folacin	Green vegetables Whole grains and dry beans Organ meats (also B_6, B_{12})	To help enzyme and other biochemical systems function normally
Vitamin C Ascorbic Acid	Citrus fruits (lemons, oranges, grapefruit, limes) Strawberries, cantaloupe Tomatoes Green peppers, broccoli Raw or lightly cooked greens Cabbage White potatoes	To make cementing materials that hold body cells together To make firm blood-vessel walls To help resist infection To help prevent fatigue To help in healing wounds and broken bones

(Cont. on p. 54)

Nutrient	Important Food Sources	Use in the Body
Vitamin D (Sunshine Vitamin)	Vitamin D milk Butter Fish-liver oil Sunshine (not a food!)	To help the body absorb calcium from digestive tract To help build calcium and phosphorus into bones
Calcium	Milk Cheese, especially Cheddar-type Ice cream Turnip and mustard greens Collards, kale, broccoli Canned sardines, salmon	To help build bones, teeth To help make blood clot To help muscles react normally To delay fatigue and help tired muscles recover
Iodine	Seafoods Iodized salt	To make thyroxine, an essential hormone that regulates metabolic rate To prevent (simple) goiter
Iron	Liver Meat and eggs Green leafy vegetables Raisins, dried apricots	To combine with protein to make hemoglobin, the red substance in the blood that carries oxygen to the cells

7

Vitamin-Mineral Supplements

Happiness is not a destination, but the pulse of life.
On menu of "The Laughing Man"
Restaurant in Nashville, Tennessee

It has been said that 10 percent of the people in this country are anemic and 25 percent are overweight, and that over half of the population does not eat well enough to be classified as even enjoying life. Actually, when you look around, you may be inclined to doubt that those percentages are quite accurate. If you scan the magazines, you will note that almost every one of them has a feature article dealing with the subject of being overweight. The figure of 25 percent may be a gross underestimate.

If that many people are overweight, why all the fuss about nutrition and vitamins and food supplements? How healthy do overweight people look to you? People are *not* overweight because they are overnourished! Quite the contrary.

Let's Dispel Some Myths

Many people have backed off from an investigation of good nutrition because they have been turned off by a lot of erroneous information that has been spread around for years. The implication is that health-conscious individuals are faddists, quacks, or some kind of counterculture food nuts. Dr. J. F. Montague has made the observation that when life hangs by a thread, people are sorry they didn't take a health "stitch in time."

Resistance to thinking about these matters of better nutrition is breaking down. Some of the strongest defenders and loudest exponents for a return to eating "nature's way" are

55

young men and women. That is a healthy sign, due in some measure to their observations of the breakdown in health of their parents and other adults. Abuse of health sometimes doesn't show up for twenty to thirty years.

Certainly one of the reasons the message of this book and others like it is so vital is the indisputable fact that our children and teenagers are only building future misery for themselves if they do not now confront the weight of accumulated evidence that proves that Americans do not eat nutritiously.

You do need to work at this matter of providing nutritional meals for yourself and/or your family. There are many options available to the creative individual who is willing to invest and expend the time necessary to seek out ways and means for doing this very thing.

There *is* hope—and while vitamins and food supplements are by no means a cure-all that will spell instant health and mean health insurance, enough evidence exists to warrant an open-minded investigation. The best approach is to use supplements and give yourself a chance to cultivate the taste for as many foods as you can tolerate that are nutritionally superior.

Why did biblical man live for as long as he did? Why do people like the Hunzas, living high in the Himalayas, have such good health? The food of the Hunza people is limited, but statistics on their longevity and good health are a matter of documentation. The Hunza people have no ulcers, cancers, heart or kidney diseases—or other illnesses such as are common to civilized modern man. Their cheerfulness and endurance are incredible.

We can find natives in Central Africa, South America, and parts of Mexico who are free from the diseases and problems that plague us in this country. Statistics don't tell the whole story, but the answer to the *why* relates directly to *what* they are eating and drinking. In stark contrast to these so-called primitive peoples, we in this country lead the world in the number of deaths from heart disease and cancer. Strokes, high blood pressure, emphysema, diabetes, and other degenerative diseases are increasing rapidly.

For Total Well-being

The writer of Proverbs says: "A wise man is strong; yea, a man of knowledge increaseth strength" (Proverbs 24:5 KJV). We are inclined to apply that to everything but our physical well-being. Who is to say that the reason we *are not* so strong, healthy and disease-free is that our eating habits are so dreadfully far amiss from what the Creator intended them to be!

The moral, ethical, and spiritual precepts outlined for us throughout the Bible are there for our *total* well-being. For instance, we are told: "When thou sittest to eat . . . consider diligently what is before thee: And put a knife to thy throat, if thou be a man given to appetite. Be not desirous of his dainties: for they are deceitful meat" (Proverbs 23:1–3 KJV).

What could be more plain?

Researchers cannot use human beings as guinea pigs; they use animals. Time after time it has been proven that a faulty diet can produce certain deficiencies and diseases in animals. Disease in humans is going to come about in exactly the same way as it is produced in laboratory animals—by inadequate diets!

The Silent Violence in Food

We have not even touched on the problems of additives in our foods, nor the controversy this has kicked up in recent years. Millions of people were jolted out of their complacency when Jacqueline Verrett, a leading scientist with the Food and Drug Administration, and Jean Carper, a freelance writer specializing in consumer health subjects, wrote the book *Eating May Be Hazardous to Your Health.* Ralph Nader stated: "This is a soberly gripping book . . . . The story they tell about the silent violence in your food—how it got there and the FDA's abysmal lack of courage to make the food companies obey the law—makes you want to do something about it."

The gist of the book by these two women was that notwithstanding the FDA's proclamations to the contrary, all is not right with our food supply, and we had best do something about it. They make the disturbing observation that we have more free choice about drugs than about the food chemicals we eat.

Biochemical Suffocation

The oft-quoted and much-respected Dr. Roger Williams commented on this very serious situation in an article which appeared in *American Laboratory* (April 1974). He asked, "How do people get perfect nutrition—every item in just the right amount?" Then he answered by stating, "They don't." His explanation was that people get along on imperfect nutrition just as corn plants growing in a field and producing ten bushels an acre instead of two hundred bushels, which is possible. Dr. Williams states that a perfect food environment is as rare as a perfect climatic environment. He points out that just one of the reasons why we need good nutrition is to feed not only our bodies, but our brains.

Good Nutrition Is Preventive Medicine

We need to think of good nutrition as preventive medicine. This might take some of the controversial aspects of the matter out of the way and allow us to look at the subject from a different standpoint.

While it is always wise to consult with one's doctor before embarking on any major new diet plan (particularly for extremely overweight people), we have to recognize that most physicians are not experts in nutrition. We would never underestimate their expertise in areas of diagnosing illness, administration of drugs, and performing surgical procedures, but doctors themselves (for the most part) would admit that they are not specifically trained regarding nutrition. This is not to belittle their profession; it is simply to acknowledge that they are trained to treat illness, save lives and relieve pain, that few of them are taught how to *prevent* illness.

We are to be guardians of our own health and the well-being of those children God has entrusted to us. The Prophet Hosea cried out as the Lord gave him utterance: "My people are destroyed for lack of knowledge . . ." (Hosea 4:6 KJV).

The destruction in human lives—the misery and heartache that are endured by countless millions—is justifiable cause to rise up and be counted and reutter the prophet's words, albeit in a different context.

Who Needs Vitamins and Supplements?

The need for vitamins and other diet supplements has been proven for many types of people in various situations.

Dieters should realize that many vital nutrients are often eliminated when an individual becomes serious about weight reduction.

Women on birth-control pills may need the B-complex vitamins in particular—and vitamin C.

Pregnant women discover that most gynecologists immediately prescribe vitamin–mineral supplements for their patients. Pregnancy creates a greater demand than ever for all vital nutrients.

In addition, women in the work force, whose hectic schedules give little time for serious meal planning; people who live alone and tend to skip or skimp on meals; and older people, living on limited funds, would do well to include food supplements. Smokers should be aware that many vitamins are destroyed by smoking and that vitamins A, E, and C may be needed. Deficiencies may also develop for people with prolonged illnesses or for those taking medication for heart disorders, diabetes, epilepsy, and drug addiction. Special note should be given to children and teenagers, athletes, hard workers, formula-fed infants, the poor, the rich, and those who lead sedentary lives.

When should vitamin–mineral supplements be taken? Before or *during* each meal, when digestive juices are flowing. It is better to divide the number you take, so that you have them three times a day for maximum benefit. If you do it this way, you will insure having *all* the essential nutrients present at the same time in your digestive tract. This is essential for optimal growth, maintenance, and repair of your body and brain cells.

Use common sense in taking vitamin–mineral supplements. "A little is good, so a whole lot is better," is simply not true. The treatment of disease should be in the hands of those skilled in diagnosis and treatment, but supplements designed to prevent, or to help serve as insurance against the development of nutritional deficiencies are available to us. We can make our own decisions regarding the use of them.

The Apostle Peter cautioned: "Be sober, be vigilant; because your adversary the devil, as a roaring lion, walketh about, seeking whom he may devour" (1 Peter 5:8 KJV). You may not apply that to the need to be alert and on the watch regarding what you eat and what goes into your body, but we do. The devil is a destroyer. He has been from the very beginning, and we have been lax and remiss in our failure to recognize the fact that one of the weapons he has used with great success is food!

If health was a thing that money could buy,
The rich would live and the poor would die;
But God in His wisdom has willed it so:
Obey Nature's laws or live in pain and woe.

ANONYMOUS

8

Action Line for Good Nutrition

Man has sought the elixir of life and has pursued the
vague promise of lasting youth or immortality since
the beginning of time . . . . The keys to the well-
guarded secrets of longevity may well turn out to be
a combination of interacting causes. Emotional
poise, balanced nutrition and favorable environment are just some of the basic elements of a long
and satisfying life. No one isolated item can suffice
in maintaining perfect health. We must pursue an
intelligent course of action which is possible only
through a better knowledge of what our bodies
need.

Bernard Jensen
World Keys to Health and Long Life

What can be done to improve our food, so that we can depend upon it to supply our needs? Nutritional travesties have
been foisted upon the gullible American public for longer
than most of us can remember. It took those crusaders who
were labeled "food faddists" to finally wake up enough
people so that some measures have been taken.

Watchdogs of Nutrition

You run a nutritional obstacle course as a concerned
homemaker when you try to set before your family everything
that they need for super-great nutrition. In this country we
have three federal agencies which act as the watchdogs of the
food industry: the Food and Drug Administration (FDA), the
United States Department of Agriculture (USDA), and the
Federal Trade Commission (FTC). Our food supply is gener-

ally considered to be bacterially safe. It certainly is, for the
most part, abundant in quantity.

In spite of this, the National Health Education Committee
lists these ten diseases as affecting the greatest portion of the
American population:

1. Heart and circulatory disorders
2. Allergic disorders
3. Mental and emotional disorders
4. Arthritis and rheumatic diseases
5. Hearing impairments
6. Mental retardation
7. Visual disturbances
8. Diabetes mellitus
9. Neurological disorders
10. Cancer

Dr. Edith Weir, of the USDA, reported in August 1971 that
many health benefits would result from better nutrition. Up to
300,000 lives could be saved from heart disease and stroke
each year, and 150,000 lives could be saved from cancer.
Death rates for unborn children, infants, and mothers giving
birth could be cut in half. The 250 million cases of respiratory
infections causing 80,000 deaths each year could be reduced
by 20 percent. Substantial reductions would occur in mental
illness, arthritis, allergies, alcoholism, dental problems, diabetes, digestive ailments, blindness, kidney disease, muscular
disorders, and obesity. Improvements would occur in life-
span, learning ability, and personal appearance.

What are you going to do so that you and your family don't
end up as statistics on lists such as this? According to Dr. E.
Cheraskin (chief of the Department of Oral Medicine of the
University of Alabama), ". . . if the present rate of increase of
sickness in this country keeps up, one may expect all persons
now 17–24 years old to be ill by 1997. I would suspect that this
would be largely a function of dietary intake." And that projec-
tion is for only one age group!

Positive Things You Can Do

1. Support national food labeling, so we will know what is in the food we eat.

2. Urge the canning of fruits in their own juices or water pack, rather than in heavy syrup.

3. Urge that dried fruits be dipped in a vitamin-C solution to prevent oxidation and darkening, rather than in a sulfur solution.

4. Urge the use of vitamin E in foods to prevent the oxidation that allows fatty foods to become rancid, rather than BHT and BHA.

5. Tax carbonated soft drinks. Educate your children against the use of them.

6. Emphasize the use of foods as they come from the field, orchard, and dairy, rather than overprocessed foods.

7. Eliminate sugar-rich foods.

8. Discourage the marketing of more new convenience foods, which contain very little natural foods—by law, if necessary.

9. Lobby for a law to be passed preventing processing of grains and the loss of valuable nutrients. Some countries have done this and greatly improved the health of the people.

10. Eat less animal fats, as these saturated fats are a contributing cause of arteriosclerosis (*see* Leviticus 3:17 and 7:22–24). How can we avoid eating a lot of animal fat when it is marbled through our meat due to the unnatural breeding for greater fat on our cattle and hogs? Some of us have discovered other ways to receive our protein.

11. Understand God's provision for keeping the land fertile as given in Leviticus 25:3–5. There was no need for chemical fertilizers when this rule was followed, as the land was able to retain its fertility.

12. Make use of a supply of calcium in bone meal available to us through our huge meat-processing plants. Americans as a whole are calcium deficient, since we depend almost entirely on milk products for our calcium. Many foods should be fortified with bone meal, as we do our animal foods (our animals

are better fed than our people). Egg shells and oyster shells are also good sources of calcium. They are mostly waste products now.

13. Encourage the fortification of more foods with protein, vitamins, and minerals. We prefer to see people eat more natural foods, but if they insist on eating junk or empty-calorie foods, then even some of the junk foods should be fortified.

14. Last, we must ever keep in mind that we live in an imperfect world. "For we know that the whole creation groaneth and travaileth in pain together until now . . ." (Romans 8:22 KJV). We cannot expect to have perfect health, but we can try to do everything possible to maintain fairly good health.

The charts at the end of this chapter picture the contrasts between the typical *inadequate* American diet and one that is considered *adequate*—with the same number of calories.

And What Are You Drinking?

"Water can feed or destroy us, leeching the soil and carrying away chemicals necessary for a balanced body. Yet the largest part of our body is made up of water, and the purity of this water is necessary for long life."

Water is second only to oxygen in importance to the vital needs of the human body. An adult needs from two to two and one-half quarts a day in the form of fluid foods and drinking water. The normal person takes into his body about a ton of water each year.

Water accounts for between 55 and 65 percent of total body weight. Your blood is 90 percent water.

One of the primary functions of water in the body is to act as a solvent; i.e., it transports nutrients to the various cells of the body and also removes the cellular waste products. What a fantastic system the Lord has put into the complex body of man!

Nature's Way of Perpetuity

The Bible speaks of seeds as being "precious" (Psalms 126:6). There are numerous references to seeds in the Word of God, and they refer to life processes. One of the most beautiful of such references is found in Isaiah 55:10, 11: "As the rain and snow come down from heaven and stay upon the ground to water the earth, and cause the grain to grow and to produce seed for the farmer and bread for the hungry, so also is my Word. I send it out and it always produces fruit. It shall accomplish all I want it to, and prosper everywhere I send it."

At the outset of this book we pointed out how God, at the time of Creation, said: ". . . Let the earth burst forth with every sort of grass and seed-bearing plant, and fruit trees with seeds inside the fruit, so that these seeds will produce the kinds of plants and fruits they came from" (Genesis 1:11).

Are you eating seeds? You should be. There is high nutritive value in seeds. They definitely are the highest protein food in the vegetable kingdom, containing nearly all the ten essential amino acids. Seeds help to take the place of meat, thereby providing essential protein for our bodies. The Hunzas claim the apricot seed is partly responsible for their long lives. You will want to get acquainted with sesame seeds, sunflower seeds and pumpkin seeds, in particular.

Nuts: The Perfect Meat Substitute

Nuts are tasty, handy to eat, and good for you. Eaten fresh from the shell, they are easier to digest than if toasted in oil. Nuts provide high-quality protein. They contain much iron and a high content of calcium and are available in a wide variety.

Typical American Diet (Inadequate)

Food	Calories	Protein	Fat	Carbohydrate	Calcium	Iron	Vit. A	Thiamine	Riboflavin	Niacin	Ascorbic Acid
Breakfast											
Cornflakes ½ c.	55	2		12	2	.2		.06	.01	.3	2
Canned pears (syrup) ½ c.	100			25	7	.3		.02	.03	.2	1
Milk ⅓ c.	50	3	3	4	96		117	.03	.14		
Sugar 2 tsp.	30			8							
White toast 2 sl.	120	4	2	24	32	.4		.04	.04	.6	
Margarine 1 Tbsp.	100		11				460				
Coffee 2 tsp. sugar	30			8							
Coffee Break											
Coffee 2 tsp. sugar	30			8							
Doughnut	125	1	6	16	13	.4	30	.05	.05	.4	
Lunch											
Cr. of mushroom soup 1 c.	135	2	10	10	41	.5	70	.02	.12	.7	
Crackers 4	70	2	2	12	4	.2					
Plain gel. 1 c.	140	4		34							
Plain cookies 2	240	2	10	36	18	.4	40	.02	.02	.2	
Coffee Break											
Coke 1 c.	95			24							
Plain cookies 2	240	2	10	36	18	.4	40	.02	.02	.2	
Dinner											
Roast beef 3 oz.	375	17	34		8	2.2	70	.05	.13	3.1	
Fr. fried potatoes	155	2	7	20	9	.7	40	.07	.04	1.8	12
Beets	50	2		12	23	.8		.04	.07	.5	11
Lettuce, mayonnaise	120	1	12		37	.8	990	.03	.05	.2	9
Cake	370	4	14	59	63	.6	180	.02	.09	.2	
Total	2630	48	121	348	371	7.9	2037	.47	.81	8.4	35
Recommended (male 35-55)	2600	65			800	10.0	5000	1.30	1.70	17.0	60

Note: Although this is a typical American diet, it is deficient in everything except calories. It would be impossible to maintain good health on such a diet.

Typical American Diet (Adequate)

Food	Calories	Protein	Fat	Carbohydrate	Calcium	Iron	Vit. A	Thiamine	Riboflavin	Niacin	Ascorbic Acid
Breakfast											
Orange juice ½ c.	110	2		27	22	.2	500	.21	.03	.8	112
Boiled eggs 2	160	13	12	1	54	2.3	1180	.09	.28	.1	
Whole wheat toast 2 sl.	110	4	2	22	46	1.0		.12	.06	1.4	
Margarine 1 Tbsp.	100		11		3		469				
Coffee Break											
Decaf. coffee (no sugar)											
2 Tbsp. milk	20	1	1	2	38		90	.01	.05		
Cheddar cheese											
2 slices	140	8	10		256	.4	440		.16		
Crackers 4	70	2	2	12	4	.2					
Lunch											
Vegetable beef soup 1 c.	80	5	2	10	12	.7	2700	.05	.05	1.0	
Crackers 4	70	2	2	12	4	.2					
Margarine 1 Tbsp.	100		11		3		469				
Gelatin with fruit	220	3		50	15	.4	120	.20	.06	.5	17
Oatmeal cookies	170	3	3	32	23	.7	40	.07	.03	.5	
Hot chocolate	235	9	11	26	286	.9	390	.09	.45	.4	2
Dinner											
Hamburger patty 3 oz.	245	21	17		9	2.7	30	.07	.18	4.6	
Baked potato	90	3		21	9	.7		.10	.04	1.7	20
Margarine 2 Tbsp.	200		22		6		938				
Peas	115	9	1	19	37	2.9	860	.44	.17	3.7	33
Cole slaw	120	1		9	52	.5	180	.06	.06	.3	35
Whole wheat bread 2 sl.	110	4	2	22	46	1.0		.12	.06	1.4	
Ice cream	145	3	9	15	87	.1	370	.03	.13	.1	1
Total	2610	93	139	280	1012	14.9	8776	1.66	1.81	16.5	220
Recommended (male 35-55)	2600	65			800	10.0	5000	1.30	1.70	17.0	60

Note: This diet is adequate in all respects, even though the calories are about the same as in the previous chart. The difference lies in the foods which were chosen. It is not a faddist diet, but could be considered a typical one for Americans.

9

Help for the Overweight

I keep my health by dieting. People gorge themselves with rich foods, use up their time, ruin their
digestion and poison themselves. If the doctors
would prescribe dieting instead of drugs, the ailments of normal man would disappear. Half the
people are food drunk all the time. Dieting is my
secret of health.

Thomas Edison

Habitual moderation means not overdoing, not going to ex-
tremes, not indulging oneself in excessive appetites. Some
call it temperance, the most important key to good health and
longevity.

No book on food and nutrition would be complete without a
chapter on the problems of being overweight. Why is this such
a problem? Why is being overweight steadily on the increase?
There are many possible reasons:

1. We have an abundance of food, so we eat for the pleasure
of eating.

2. Coffee breaks encourage people to snack between meals.

3. People snack while watching television.

4. We live in a mechanical age. Machinery does much of
our work for us; the automobile has replaced walking. Our
pioneer ancestors could eat twice as much as we do and still
not put on weight, because they worked it off.

5. Eating is often a part of our socializing: i.e., potluck dinners in church, banquets, luncheons, and so on.

6. People eat to make up for loneliness and unhappiness; it
is one way to assuage grief. Eating seems to be a way to gratify
emotional needs.

The Key

The key to weight loss is to keep the caloric intake at a level that requires the body to turn to its storehouse of fat for the energy it needs. Losing pounds requires that you burn up more calories than you consume.

We have seen many individuals give up in despair when the hoped-for weight loss didn't come right away. It is unrealistic to expect that this will happen immediately. Remember, you didn't put that excess weight on overnight—more than likely it is an accumulation acquired over a matter of years.

Give your body time to adjust, give yourself *plenty* of time, but hang in there and it will come off. Just how long you'll have to stay with a diet plan depends on how much you need to lose. Once you reach that desired goal, if you have trained yourself to think of health, you won't have any trouble staying right where you want to be. For one thing, you are going to feel so much better, and look so great, you'll never allow yourself to fall backwards again.

Are You a Mental Overweight?

There are some people who say they have a weight problem, but in reality the problem exists only from the neck up—in the head! These are the individuals (especially true among women) who annoy everyone by their attempts to attain an unreasonable slimness, an ideal they have in their heads that is not only unattainable, but downright unhealthy.

They are "mental overweights"—they have fallen victim to what is called the skinny-model syndrome, and have allowed themselves to be unreasonably influenced by the TV commercials and fashion magazines. Unnecessary crash dieting is foolish. A preoccupation with your weight will sap creative energy, take the joy out of living, and make life miserable for others around you. It could result in an unwise compromise on your part in the matter of health and nutrition.

So much has been written on the subject of weight control. Our approach may not be new; but we hope that it will provide new motivation to help you get started.

Bernard Jensen found that healthy elderly people had one

thing in common: They ate very little, had small meals, and many of them had only one meal a day. When they did eat, portions were always small. As Benjamin Franklin said, "To lengthen thy life, lessen thy meals."

God has created us with economy in our bodies. The Apostle Paul said, for good reason, "Let your moderation be known unto all men" (Philippians 4:5 KJV). Elsewhere he uses the illustration of the well-known Greek games to illustrate the spiritual race of the unbeliever. He says:

> In a race, everyone runs but only one person gets first prize. So run your race to win. To win the contest you must deny yourselves many things that would keep you from doing your best. An athlete goes to all this trouble just to win a blue ribbon or a silver cup, but we do it for a heavenly reward that never disappears. So I run straight to the goal with purpose in every step. I fight to win. I'm not just shadow-boxing or playing around.
>
> 1 Corinthians 9:24–26

Paul continues with the illustration, telling the reader that he keeps his body under subjection.

We take that and apply it to our spiritual lives, and rightly so. All of this has reference to living what, in Christian circles, we call the abundant life. Dynamic, abundant living is not just for a few—it's God's norm for all believers. But we believe that this kind of living will be greatly enhanced if you are not only feeling, but looking, better. And that has a lot to do with what you are putting into your physical body as well as what you may be giving your spiritual body.

Longer Waistline, Shorter Lifeline

It goes almost without saying that being overweight presents a hazard to health and long life. Overweight people are much more susceptible to chronic diseases such as diabetes, high-blood pressure, heart conditions, and so on.

Although Americans are obsessed with losing weight and spend over four million dollars a year for reducing drugs and treatments, some people have been on every known kind of diet and are still overweight. Not only do they have flabby flesh, but the root cause of all their troubles is that they have flabby willpower.

Dr. Stanley Mooneyham, in his book *What Do You Say to a Hungry World?*, points out that most Americans generally eat 900 more calories than they need and twice as much protein as their bodies can use. He says that one restaurant in this country wastes two and one-half tons of meat and one quarter ton of butter in one year. He shows how it takes twenty-one pounds of protein feed (soybeans, and so on) to produce one pound of protein in steak. These and other facts are terribly sobering. They should provide an impetus to the overweight reader to do something *right now* about his or her obvious problem.

Recognition must come that we have got to give our bodies a new beginning if we are going to get out of this awful predicament of being overweight. Where does one begin? You begin by learning the new ways of attaining and then maintaining good health. Dieting has become a way of life to the average American. Maybe you need to get off a diet, stop thinking about dieting, and start thinking of learning a good healthy way to live.

Biochemical Reactions Involved

People can be divided into two groups according to the way their bodies deal with the excess food they eat. An experiment was conducted in which a scientist took people whose weights had been constant over the years, and had them eat double and treble their normal amount of food. They did not put on weight. They responded to overeating by increasing their metabolic rate (rate of using up food), and thus burned up the extra calories. He then overfed people whose weights had not remained constant in the past, and found that they showed no increase in metabolism, but put on weight. We all know people who can eat large amounts of food but do not gain weight, while others gain weight on a small amount of food.

The above has been proven to be true in the last ten to fifteen years. Research has revealed the biochemical reactions which go on in the body. Details of the metabolism of fats, carbohydrates, and proteins have been clarified and new information gained. It has been found that the carbohydrate foods (starches and sugars) are what cause weight gain, because the person who fattens easily has a defective capacity for dealing with carbohydrates. Excess carbohydrate is deposited as fat, rather than being used for energy and heat. This inability to deal with carbohydrate is due to a block in the chain of chemical reactions leading from glucose to the release of heat and energy.

The chemical reactions which enable the body to deal with food can go wrong. They depend on certain hormones and enzymes, which some people lack or are unable to manufacture properly. The trouble is thought to be their inability to oxidize pyruvic acid, and this is bad for them in two ways: They cannot use carbohydrate for energy, so they deposit it as fat; and it prevents the breakdown of their own body fat by inhibiting the oxidation of fatty acids. By eating mostly fat and protein, they by-pass their metabolic block.

There has been criticism of the high-protein, high-fat diet, in that it can lead to ketosis (an end product of fat metabolism). There are degrees of ketosis, and the effects of the severe ketosis of diabetes are quite different from those of the mild ketosis of a fasting person, or the even milder ketosis of a person on a high-fat diet. There may even be possible advantages of ketosis to the obese, as the benign ketosis which develops when carbohydrates are in short supply increases the mobilization of stored body fat for fuel and assists weight loss.

The foods in the Basic Four food groups can be adapted to a reducing diet:

Milk group—2 glasses skim milk or buttermilk
Meat group—3 or more servings
Vegetable and fruit group—6 or more servings
Bread and cereal group—1 serving
Fat—2 tablespoons of oil or soft margarine
Sugar and sweets—none

We have included below "The Weight-Reducer's Diet," developed for use in weight-reduction clinics in connection with a local public-health department. It spells out what foods can be eaten and which ones are absolute don'ts. It also contains menu plans, suggestions, and recipes.

A study of the Bible seems to indicate very strongly that fasting was the method used to keep weight down in biblical days. Two days of fasting each week would surely be instrumental in preventing weight gain above normal, and also bring about other health benefits.

The Weight-Reducer's Diet

Basic Rules

There is no need to count calories, but you should weigh or measure foods as indicated.

Never skip a meal.

Do not add or subtract foods from the diet lists as given.

Eat As Desired the Following Foods:

Beverages

Water
Natural fruit juices
Bouillon and clear soups (fat free)
Herb tea or decaffeinated coffee (no sugar)
One cup of tomato juice

Seasonings and sauces

All spices and herbs	Horseradish
Vinegar	Salt and pepper
Mustard	Unflavored gelatin

Low-calorie vegetables

Asparagus	Green pepper
Bean sprouts	Lettuce, endive, watercress
Broccoli	Mushrooms
Cabbage, sauerkraut	Spinach, parsley, other greens
Cauliflower	String beans
Celery	Summer squash, zucchini
Cucumber	

Higher-calorie vegetables: ½ cup or four oz. daily

Beets   Onions
Brussels sprouts   Peas, lima beans
Carrots, parsnips, turnips   Winter squash, pumpkin
Okra

Fruits

Eat three fruits every day, one a vitamin-C fruit, such as oranges or grapefruit. Fruits may be fresh, water- or diet-packed, canned or frozen, unsweetened.

Berries, ½ cup
Orange or grapefruit juice (unsweetened), ½ cup
Medium-sized pineapple, ¼
Medium-sized grapefruit, ½
Medium-sized cantaloupe, ½
Honeydew or other melon, one-inch wedge
Do not eat bananas, cherries, grapes, dried fruits, tropical fruits.

Meat, fish, poultry

Broil, bake, or roast—do not fry. Remove all visible fat before cooking and/or eating. Do not eat gravies or sauces.

Fish, oysters, clams, crabs, shrimp
Beef, veal, lamb, chicken, turkey, venison, rabbit
Eat fish several times a week, liver once a week.

Eggs, cheese, and fats

One egg daily, cooked any way but fried.
Cottage cheese and hard cheese (American, Swiss, Jack, etc.)
Diet margarine or oil, 2 Tbsp.

Milk

Skim milk or buttermilk, two eight-ounce glasses daily. Suggest using eight ounces of plain yogurt in place of one glass of milk.

Bread

Whole wheat bread, one slice for breakfast daily.

Absolute Don'ts

Alcoholic beverages
Bacon
Butter or plain margarine
Cake, cookies, crackers, pie
Candy, chocolate, coconut
Cereals, breakfast foods
Cream, sweet or sour
Ice cream, frozen desserts
Mayonnaise, salad dressings
Dried beans and peas
Muffins, biscuits, doughnuts
Pancakes, waffles

Nuts, peanut butter
Pork products
Potatoes, p. chips, pretzels
Puddings, custards,
    flavored gelatin
Rice, corn, catsup
Rolls, special breads
Smoked fish, meats, luncheon meats
Spaghetti, macaroni, noodles
Sweetened soda pops
Sugar, syrups, honey, jams

Suggested Menu Plans

Breakfast

Orange or grapefruit juice (½ cup), or ½ grapefruit or cantaloupe or other fruit
One egg, or one ounce hard cheese, or two ounces fish, or ¼ cup cottage cheese
One slice whole-wheat toast with ½ tsp. fortified butter
Beverage

Snack

One glass skim milk, or one cup yogurt, or one cup tomato juice

Lunch

Three to four ounces fish, lean meat, or poultry, or ⅔ cup cottage cheese, or two ounces hard cheese, or two eggs
Any amount of low-calorie vegetables
½ cup fruit

Snack
One glass skim milk, or one cup yogurt, or one cup tomato juice

Dinner
Four to six ounces lean meat, fish, poultry, or liver
½ cup (four ounces) cooked higher-calorie vegetable with one tsp. diet margarine
Any amount of low-calorie vegetables
½ cup fruit
Beverage

Breakfast
½ grapefruit
One soft-boiled egg
One slice whole-wheat toast with ½ tsp. fortified butter
One cup herb tea or black coffee

Snack
One glass skim milk

Lunch
Three to four ounces canned tuna
Salad of lettuce, celery, and radishes with diet dressing
½ cup fresh peaches
Tea

Snack
One cup plain tomato juice

Dinner
Four to six ounces liver
½ cup peas with ½ tsp. fortified butter
½ cup apple sauce
One glass skim milk

Breakfast
½ cup orange juice
One slice American cheese on one slice whole-wheat bread
with ½ tsp. fortified butter
One cup coffee (if you must; herb tea recommended)

Snack
One cup plain yogurt

Lunch
1½ cups oyster stew made with three ounces oysters and
one cup skim milk and ½ tsp. fortified butter
One cup broccoli
½ cup diet-packed canned pears

Snack
One cup tomato juice

Dinner
Four to six ounces ground beef
½ cup yellow squash with ½ tsp. fortified butter
One cup tossed salad with diet dressing
½ cup fresh strawberries or unsweetened frozen

Weight-Reducer Recipes

French Toast
One egg, beaten
Two Tbsp. skim milk
One slice whole-wheat bread
*Soak bread in mixture of egg and skim milk. Broil on
aluminum foil until brown on one side. Turn over and brown
other side.*

Soda Milk Shake
½ cup diet soda (any flavor)
One cup skim milk
Six ice cubes
Put all ingredients in blender. Beat until frothy and thick.

Fruit Milk Shake
½ cup any fruit (berries, peaches, apples, etc.)
One cup skim milk
Honey to sweeten
Six ice cubes
Put all ingredients in blender. Beat until frothy and thick.

Diet French Dressing
One cup tomato juice
½ cup vinegar
½ tsp. dry mustard
¼ tsp. garlic salt and onion salt
Honey to sweeten

Quick Hollandaise Sauce
One cup buttermilk or plain yogurt
½ tsp. lemon juice
¼ tsp. salt
½ tsp. dry mustard
Honey to sweeten slightly, if desired

10

Should One Fast?

Abstinence and quiet cure many diseases . . . .

Hippocrates

Fasting is nothing new; although much more is being made of the practice these days than in the past. Authors of new fasting books are loudly touting its praises as the quickest, easiest way possible to lose weight. Such authors consider fasting to be "the ultimate diet." What they are saying is quite literally true—but fasting for the sake of losing weight—and extending the practice over a considerable period of time—is not wise unless you have first consulted with your family doctor.

There are some individuals who should not fast. This would include expectant and nursing mothers, diabetics who are taking insulin, and people with terminal illness. Children should not fast unless medically supervised. But fasting needs our consideration, as a practice that will yield physical benefits and provide great spiritual enrichment.

Famous Fasters

Old Testament examples of fasting are Moses (Exodus 34:28), the children of Israel (Judges 20:26), Elijah (1 Kings 19:8), David and his men (2 Samuel 1:12), the valiant men of Jabesh-gilead (1 Chronicles 10:12), King Jehoshaphat (2 Chronicles 20:3), Ezra (Ezra 8:21), Nehemiah (Nehemiah 1:4), Esther, her uncle, and the Jews in Shushan (Esther 4:16), David (Psalms 35:13; 109:24), Daniel (Daniel 9:3; 10:3), Joel called for a fast (Joel 1:14), the people of Nineveh (Jonah 3:5–7).

New Testament examples include Jesus (Matthew 4:2; Luke

4:2), the disciples of John, and the Pharisees (Matthew 9:14, 15). Jesus' teachings concerning fasting can be found in Matthew 17:21; Mark 2:18–20; Mark 9:29; Luke 5:33–35. Paul experienced and taught the value of fasting in Acts 9:9; 13:2; 14:23; 27:33; 1 Corinthians 7:5; 2 Corinthians 6:5; 11:27. Also note Cornelius (Acts 10:30). There are other references to fasting, but these are the most familiar examples from the Bible.

There have been famous fasters in history. Hippocrates, an outstanding physician of his time (born about 460 B.C.), advocated abstinence from food for health reasons. What did Hippocrates believe? Simply that nature was the principal healer, and that fasting was beneficial to the body. It was his belief that the more we nourish unhealthy bodies, the more we injure them. He advocated eating only one meal a day.

Great Christian leaders such as Luther, Wesley, Calvin, and Knox fasted, as did the American Indians, the Puritans, and Benjamin Franklin. Gandhi of India was known for his fasts. Novelist Upton Sinclair fasted often during his ninety years, and entertainer Dick Gregory made headlines with his fasts. Many other examples could be cited. The evidence is overwhelmingly clear—fasting is a practice that yields benefits.

Spiritual Benefits

1. Fasting is a discipline of the body in order to humble the soul. David said: "I chastened my soul with fasting . . ." (Psalms 69:10 KJV).

2. Fasting helps prevail in prayer with God. "So we fasted and besought our God for this: and he was intreated of us" (Ezra 8:23 KJV). When we are willing to set aside the appetites of the body to concentrate on prayer, it demonstrates that we mean business.

3. Fasting with prayer may bring mercy from God, rather than judgment. "[The Lord says:] '. . . Turn to me now, while there is time. Give me all your hearts. Come with fasting, weeping, mourning. Let your remorse tear at your hearts and not your garments.' Return to the Lord your God, for he is gracious and merciful . . ." (Joel 2:12, 13).

4. Fasting may free us from weaknesses of the flesh such as smoking, drinking, drugs, unnatural sexual desire, and even what Christians consider lesser sins, such as fears, resentment, lying, jealousy, and so on. "Is not this the fast that I have chosen? to loose the bands of wickedness, to undo the heavy burdens, and to let the oppressed go free, and that ye break every yoke?" (Isaiah 58:6 KJV).

5. Fasting may free us from bondage to Satan and give us power over him: ". . . In my name shall they cast out devils . . ." (Mark 16:17 KJV).

6. Fasting may reveal the will of God for our lives to us. It was when Peter ". . . became very hungry, and would have eaten . . ." (Acts 10:10 KJV), that God gave him the vision that led to the bringing of the Gospel to the Gentiles.

7. Fasting helps us overcome the desire for excessive amounts of food. Paul said:

> I can do anything I want to if Christ has not said no, but some of these things aren't good for me. Even if I am allowed to do them, I'll refuse to if I think they might get such a grip on me that I can't easily stop when I want to. For instance, take the matter of eating. God has given us an appetite for food and stomachs to digest it. But that doesn't mean we should eat more than we need. Don't think of eating as important, because some day God will do away with both stomachs and food.
>
> 1 Corinthians 6:12, 13

8. Fasting helps produce the fruit of the spirit—self-control (Galatians 5:22–25; 6:8; Philippians 4:5). When there is failure to deal with the lust for food, one's life is open to attack along other lines. God said of Israel, ". . . when I had fed them to the full, they then committed adultery . . ." (Jeremiah 5:7 KJV).

9. Fasting must not be allowed to degenerate into an outward form lacking spiritual value. Christ taught that fasting is a personal matter in the light of needs and circumstances. We are expected to fast, as shown by Christ's statement: ". . . Can

ye make the children of the bridechamber fast, while the bridegroom is with them? But the days will come, when the bridegroom shall be taken away from them, and then shall they fast in those days" (Luke 5:34, 35 KJV). Christ, our Bridegroom, is now taken away, and we are expected to fast.

Physical Benefits

1. Fasting is not starving, as many people think. God would not ask us to do anything harmful to our bodies. A healthy, well-nourished body can exist for several weeks without being injured or incapacitated by lack of food. Moses fasted for forty days (Exodus 34:28), and so did Elijah (1 Kings 19:8).

2. Fasting can be beneficial in the treatment of sickness and disease. Isaiah the Prophet, in describing a counterfeit fast and a true one, goes on to explain the benefits that can accrue as a result of godly fasting. He tells why God isn't impressed with the faster who continues in his oppression of others, who continues living in evil pleasure, when there is fighting and quarreling, and when his life is a lie. "This kind of fasting will never get you anywhere with me," God said through the prophet (Isaiah 58:4).

3. Fasting can bring about improvement in many chronic and acute diseases.

4. Fasting may clear up stomach ulcers by removing three sources of local irritation—the mechanical irritation brought on by particles of food in contact with the raw surface, mechanical irritation resulting from contraction and expansion of the walls of the stomach, and chemical irritation caused by acid gastric juice.

5. Fasting is a strengthener of weak hearts. The fast provides added rest for the heart, due to the lessening of the number of pulsations of the heart. Also, the reduction in weight which occurs helps, because the heart does not have to labor to keep the blood circulating through so much body bulk.

6. Fasting removes toxins and poisons from the body. The need for fasting is much greater now than it has ever been in the history of man. Air pollution in our big cities—a mixture of

soot and smoke from factories and heating plants, gaseous by-products of industry, and exhaust fumes of cars and trucks—is taken into our bodies. Our water is so filthy in many parts of the country that powerful chemicals are used to make it fit to drink. Tons of all kinds of chemicals are sprayed on our fruits and vegetables to kill harmful insects. For many years our foods have been treated with synthetic food additives that have now been discovered to be harmful to the human body. All of these foreign substances must be eliminated from the body. Fasting is the best, and perhaps the only, known way to accomplish this.

7. Fasting is the quickest, surest, safest way to lose weight. There is a safe rapid loss of weight, and hunger leaves after two or three days, so the desire to eat is missing. Weight loss will average one pound a day or more. Some physicians are now using fasting rather than dieting for reduction. Fasting will produce mild ketosis, and maintaining ketosis seems to decrease insulin's efficiency, allowing a release of fat from fat deposits.

Types of Fasts

Three types of fasting are mentioned in the Bible: the supernatural fast, the total fast, and the partial fast.

The supernatural fast is a long fast of forty days or more, in which neither food nor water is taken. Moses, Elijah, and Jesus are examples. They were supernaturally sustained by God. *We do not advise this type of fast.* The body may be able to get along without food in lengthy fasts, but not without water unless supernaturally sustained.

The total fast is going entirely without food, but includes the drinking of water. Fasts of this type may last from missing one meal to forty days or more. One fast a year, on the Day of Atonement, was all the law prescribed for the Jews. By the time of Christ, the Pharisees were observing two fasts a week. The early church by the fourth century had changed what was at first a matter of individual conscience to the practice of fasting each Wednesday and Friday. It then became only a form and a ritual. At the time of the Reformation, true fasting came back. Martin Luther, John Knox, and John Wesley practiced fasting for spiritual reasons.

The partial fast is exemplified by Daniel as stated in Daniel 10:3: "All that time I tasted neither wine nor meat, and of course I went without desserts." He fasted in this manner for three weeks and his prayers were answered. Today the partial fast is often used by beginners by the taking of juices only. This provides only a few calories, but gives necessary minerals and vitamins, and avoids the weakness and nausea sometimes present in the total fast.

How to Fast

The non-Christian may fast for physical reasons only and receive benefits, but the Christian should fast first for spiritual reasons and second, for physical benefits. Before beginning a fast we should ask ourselves: (1) Is this God's will for me at this time, and should this be a total or partial fast?; (2) What are my spiritual reasons? For personal consecration, intercession, guidance, blessing, to bring revival?; (3) Are my motives right? Is my desire for personal blessing balanced by genuine concern for others?

Set a time and start your fast. You may determine at the beginning that your fast may be for one day, three days, or even longer if the Lord leads. Or you may determine that from now on you are going to fast two days a week like the early Christians. These may be two consecutive days or separated by one or two intervening days. If at work five days a week, the weekend may be used. Some Christians get a real blessing out of fasting on Saturday and Sunday, because they are in a deep spirit of worship during church services on the second day of the fast. Do not allow yourself to be so busy on your fasting days that you cannot give time to prayer.

Breaking the Fast

After a one-day fast, normal eating may be resumed the next day. After three days or more, the fast should be broken with fruit juices, gradually adding other foods. The rule is that it should take as long to break the fast as the length of the fast was: i.e., resume normal eating the third day after a three-day fast, or the seventh day after a week's fast.

Some Important Tips

The soundest tips on fasting that we could find were in Dr. Paavo Airola's book *How to Get Well.* A summary of these rules would be:

1. *Drugs.* Complete withdrawal of drugs is advised. Exceptions would be those used for heart disease, diabetes, and arthritis. People on those drugs should have any fasting supervised by an experienced practitioner; not to do so would be most unwise.

2. *Vitamins.* Discontinue except in heart cases, very sick persons, and/or very weak patients.

3. *Smoking and drinking.* No smoking, no alcohol, and no coffee. The best way to quit smoking and drinking is by fasting!

4. *Juices.* Make them fresh and drink them immediately.

5. *Herb teas.* Peppermint, rose hips and camomile.

6. *Work.* Live your normal life and do your regular work—unless you do heavy manual-type labor—in which case, take it easy.

7. *Exercise.* To most effectively regenerate and revitalize all the body functions, do lots of walking and mild exercise in the fresh air.

8. *Daily baths.* Body impurities and wastes are eliminated through your skin; therefore, a daily shower or bath is imperative.

9. *Drinking water.* Drink to satisfy your thirst.

10. *Hunger.* Will you feel hungry? Yes, but only during the first three or four days.

11. *Positive attitude.* Your mental attitude is of paramount importance. Avoid negative influences or thoughts. Have confidence in what you are doing and tune out well-meaning friends and relatives with their warnings.

Results?

If Christians regularly followed the plan for fasting one or two days a week, not only would they be blessed spiritually, but they could avoid the problems of obesity, high blood pressure, hardening of the arteries, heart attacks, osteoarthritis, kidney stones and gallstones, and many other ills that beset modern man. It is true that we are digging our graves with our forks.

Perhaps we need to meditate upon the words of Jeremiah the Prophet as we contemplate what fasting unto the Lord could mean in our own experience from a physical and spiritual standpoint: "Your words are what sustain me; they are food to my hungry soul. They bring joy to my sorrowing heart and delight me. How proud I am to bear your name, O Lord. I have not joined the people in their merry feasts . . ." (Jeremiah 15:16–17).

11

Money Management in the Market

Eat efficiency foods instead of the deficiency foods.
Dr. Charles B. McFerrin

Where do your food dollars go? You can either save a tremendous amount of money by wise planning or throw your hard-earned dollars away. In the process, you can either give your family maximum food quality or end up giving them second best or worse. If you market with care, you can lower your expenses without sacrificing quality. Regardless of your income, wise shopping is important. We are to be good stewards of all that the Lord has given us, and it makes no difference what your income bracket is.

Dietician, artist, gracious hostess. Does that describe you? Yes, as wives and mothers we need to be gracious hostesses, and not reserve our talents along these lines just for special guests. But we need also exhibit some managerial skills, a knowledge of basic nutrition, and an understanding of the principles of food preparation.

Don't Be Penny Wise and Pound Foolish!

Try to determine the shelf life of a product. It may not be wise to buy the large economy size if you'll end up throwing part of it away because it's gone stale. This might apply when buying potatoes, cereal products, coffee, and certain perishables.

Another important consideration is your available storage. Learn to shop with your storage space in mind. Just how full is that refrigerator? Is there actually room in the freezer for the three quarts of ice cream on sale? It is false economy if you purchase more food than you can store properly.

How to Increase Your Buying Power

Practice menu planning. Use the Basic Four food plan described elsewhere in this book. Try plotting your menus for a one-week block. Take a sheet of paper and divide it into seven days, and make three columns. This will give you a block for each meal. Draw upon the information you have acquired from this book and other reading. Adapt your favorite recipes, if need be, but make certain your menus meet nutritionally acceptable standards. This may very well not only revolutionize your family's eating habits, but make your shopping excursions a real adventure.

When planning your menus, keep in mind the available time you will have for preparation.

Don't buy junk foods. Convenience foods are costly. Cook from scratch instead of buying TV dinners and packaged mixes. Compare fresh, frozen, and canned-food prices. If buying canned foods, buy house brands rather than name brands.

Shop after specials and coupons have appeared in the paper. Shop the specials, spending time at your kitchen table plotting that shopping excursion.

Stretch your milk by mixing powdered milk according to directions and then mixing it half and half with fresh milk. This brings down the cost per quart considerably.

You Can Be an Educated Shopper

Learn to judge food quality, particularly meats. It is better to purchase fresh cuts rather than prepackaged meats, if you have the choice. Always notice the ratio of meat to bone, and observe the uniformity of cut.

Buy foods in season. Not only from a budgetary standpoint is it in your own best interest to avail yourself of every seasonable opportunity to obtain certain foods, but from a health standpoint this is most beneficial. Nature is cooperating with us and trying to tell us something; we would be wise to listen.

Remember that a soft-feeling, mushy grapefruit would indicate the kind of pithiness that results when the fruit has been slightly frozen. Always notice the skin of fruits and vegetables; this is your best clue as to freshness and/or whether the produce was picked while it was too green. Skins that are shriveling a bit would be a fairly good indication that the item has begun to dehydrate and has been around too long.

To Market, to Market

The selection of where one does his marketing can make all the difference in the world in one's food budget. Comparison shopping is the name of the game in many urban areas. The shopper guides in your newspapers will provide this information. Significant savings will be yours.

Make do for the week on what you buy for that week. Dashing to the store in the middle of the week can play havoc with your food allowance. Impulse buying can wreck your budget; so can the purchase of all those nongrocery items!

You will save a considerable amount of time if you make out your grocery list according to the way your market is laid out. That isn't difficult if you shop in the same market most of the time. During the week if you run out of a grocery item, or remember that you'll need a certain item for a recipe, jot it down and keep a running list.

The Rest Is Up to You!

A doctor wise in the ways of the benefits of good nutrition has stated: "More lives can be saved for the effort expended, dollar for dollar, by getting the very best nutrition for all our people than we can ever gain with curative or preventive medicine. Creative medicine must be founded on growing and eating the best foods. Thus alone can we create real health for our people."

It is easier to plan meals when we have a pattern to go by. Following is such a pattern:

Breakfast Plan	*Example*
Fruit or fruit juice	Orange juice
Main dish	Scrambled eggs
Bread or cereal	Buttered toast
Drink	Coffee or milk

Lunch or Supper Plan	*Example*
Main dish	Tuna and noodle casserole
Vegetable and/or fruit	Lettuce and tomato salad
Bread	Whole-wheat bread
Simple dessert	Peanut butter cookies
Drink	Milk

Dinner Plan	*Example*
Main dish	Roast beef
Potatoes or alternate	Mashed potatoes
Vegetable	Buttered green beans
Salad	Cabbage and green pepper salad
Bread	Whole-wheat bread
Dessert	Custard
Drink	Lemonade

The amounts of various foods which different family members eat vary according to their size, activity, sex, and whether growth is taking place. Preschool children are growing rapidly and have small stomachs so their food must be especially nutritious. Do not allow candy and cookies to crowd out the foods needed for body building.

Teenagers need especially nourishing food, too, because of their rapid growth. Between-meal snacks are needed and should be chosen from the four food groups. Breakfast should not be omitted.

Studies have shown that calcium, vitamin A, and vitamin C are often low in the diets of the elderly. Therefore, milk, citrus fruits, and other fruits and vegetables should be emphasized in their diets.

A week's menus have been planned which incorporate these principles. The foods marked with an asterisk have recipes given for them.

A Week's Suggested Menus

Day	Breakfast	Lunch (or Supper)	Dinner
Sunday	Orange juice Creamy scrambled eggs* Whole-wheat toast Coffee, tea, or milk	Grilled cheese sandwich (whole-wheat bread) Sliced tomatoes Wheat-germ brownies * Coffee, tea, or milk	Oven-fried chicken * Baked potatoes Baked tomatoes * Tossed salad * Fruit gelatin *
Monday	Crunchy granola * Whole-wheat raisin toast Coffee, tea, or milk	Eggnog* Leftover chicken Lettuce sandwich Coffee, tea, or milk	Sautéed liver and onions* Mashed potatoes * Buttered green beans Vegetable salad * Baked cheesecake *
Tuesday	Tomato juice Whole-grain French toast with honey Coffee, tea, or milk	Cheese puff* Apple-celery salad Oatmeal cookies Coffee, tea, or milk	Bulgur meat loaf* Buttered peas Cole slaw * Wheat-germ rolls * Sliced fresh peaches
Wednesday	Cantaloupe Creamed eggs on whole-wheat toast Coffee, tea, or milk	Cottage cheese salad Sliced tomatoes Bran muffins *	Chili with beans * Cabbage cooked in milk * Corn bread Apple sauce

A Week's Suggested Menus (Cont.)

Day	Breakfast	Lunch (or Supper)	Dinner
Thursday	Prunes Cheese omelet * Rye toast Coffee, tea, or milk	Cream of corn soup Tuna sandwiches on dark bread Orange Coffee, tea, or milk	Split peas with ham * Tiny new potatoes Buttered spinach Molded carrot and pineap- ple salad Gingerbread*
Friday	Pineapple juice (with vita- min C added) Pancakes with sorghum or honey * Coffee, tea, or milk	Three-bean salad * Bran muffins * Fresh pears or other fresh fruit Coffee, tea, or milk	Baked herbed fish * Broiled ("French-fried") potatoes Green peas Tossed salad * Custard *
Saturday	Orange juice Soft-boiled eggs Bran flakes Coffee, tea, or milk	Tomato soup Peanut-butter sandwich (whole-wheat bread) Custard (from Friday) * Coffee, tea, or milk	Macaroni and cheese * Buttered zucchini Vegetable salad * Cottage cheese sherbet *

* See recipe section.

12

The Temple of the Holy Spirit

Know ye not that ye are the temple of God, and that
the Spirit of God dwelleth in you? If any man defile
the temple of God, him shall God destroy; for the
temple of God is holy, which temple ye are.

1 Corinthians 3:16, 17 KJV

If one's body is "the temple of the Holy Spirit," as the Bible
states, it is not surprising that it is likened to the Old Testament temple in many ways.

The Physical Sense

God was very zealous about His temple and often rep-
rimanded His people for their neglect of it. At times, the
people under a good leader had to clean up and repair the
temple after periods of abuse and misuse. God had intended
for His temple to be respected.

So it is with our bodies. Poor eating habits can cause illness
in ourselves and loss of respect for our bodies by others. We
should be as concerned with what we eat as we are in caring
for our outward appearance. People spend long hours better-
ing their appearance with bathing, grooming, choice of ap-
parel, and cosmetics. This is often done without giving much
attention to what we eat. We think that any food will do, as
long as it satisfies our hunger and tastes good.

Daniel of the Old Testament purposed in his heart that he
would not defile himself with the king's food and wine. He
asked for a simpler diet, and by doing so his physical appearance was far more healthy than that of others. He was blessed
by God, not only physically but spiritually. The nutritional
information set forth in this book is designed to accomplish

the same purpose. "And whatsoever ye do in word or deed, do all in the name of the Lord Jesus, giving thanks to God and the Father by him" (Colossians 3:17 KJV).

The Spiritual Sense

Spiritually, God intended the temple as a place where He met with His people to cleanse them. As God commanded the cleansing of the temple and all its objects with blood, even so we must be cleansed by the blood of Christ. ". . . without shedding of blood is no remission" (Hebrews 9:22 KJV).

The Apostle Paul prayed in 1 Thessalonians 5:23: ". . . I pray God your whole spirit and soul and body be preserved blameless unto the coming of our Lord Jesus Christ" (KJV). Paul appears to have been concerned equally about the welfare of the spirit, soul, and body.

A way of growing in spirit and soul is brought out by Paul in Philippians 4:8: ". . . whatsoever things are true, whatsoever things are honest, whatsoever things are just, whatsoever things are pure, whatsoever things are lovely, whatsoever things are of good report; if there be any virtue, and if there be any praise, think on these things" (KJV). We apply this to our spiritual lives, but in the same way we can develop a strong body by giving careful thought and study to what we should eat, and being diligent in choosing foods that will produce good health.

We must feed upon God's Word in order to grow spiritually, just as we should eat the most nourishing food in order to grow physically. Just as we are careful about doctrinal purity, we should also be careful about physical purity by eating the foods which do not harm our bodies.

God has given us an example in Esau, who thought more of his hunger than of God's blessing:

> Watch out that no one becomes . . . careless about God as Esau did: he traded his rights as the oldest son for a single meal. And afterwards, when he wanted those rights back

again, it was too late, even though he wept bitter tears of re-
pentance. So remember, and be careful.

Hebrews 12:16, 17

The temple of the Old Testament, like our bodies today,
was to be honored and respected. It was not to be defiled in
any way. The temple was never to be used as a place of
idolatry. Our bodies, therefore, are to show this single-minded
purpose of faithfulness to Christ. We must keep the inside of
the cup (our bodies) clean, as well as the outside. Spiritual
cleanliness should lead to bodily cleanliness, but too often
this is not so. What do we worship besides God? Many people
even put food before the things of God. How much better it is
to take the temple of the Holy Spirit—our body—and make it
what God intended it to be.

13

Recipes

And having food and raiment let us be therewith content.

1 Timothy 6:8 KJV

The recipes in this section put the emphasis on good nutrition rather than gourmet cooking, but the impact they will make on your family from the flavor standpoint—and their beautiful appearance—will gain for you the reputation of being a gourmet cook! By now you must be fully convinced that you and your family are going to be what you eat. We trust these recipes will help you achieve a new level of health and happiness.

The Milk Group

Milk is such an important part of our diet that we must see that the milk requirement is met, even if we have to work much of the milk into recipes. This is sometimes necessary where there are members of the family who refuse to drink milk. Concentrated forms of milk, such as evaporated milk and nonfat powdered milk, can be put into recipes. Evaporated milk may be used undiluted in custards and ice creams, and in gelatin desserts instead of whipped cream. Nonfat powdered milk may be used, not as a substitute for fresh milk, but to fortify foods. Yogurt is, of course, another nutritionally excellent form of milk. The nutritive advantages of yogurt have been emphasized elsewhere in this book.

Eggnog

1 cup fresh milk	½ tsp. salt (optional)
2 egg yolks	½ tsp. vanilla
¼ cup powdered milk	1 Tbsp. honey

Combine all ingredients and beat well, or mix in blender until smooth. For variation add fresh fruits.

Macaroni and Cheese

3 cups cooked whole-grain or enriched macaroni	1 cup evaporated milk
	1 tsp. salt
2 cups shredded cheddar cheese	¼ tsp. pepper

Preheat oven to 350°. Combine all ingredients except ½ cup of the cheese which is sprinkled on top. Bake 30 minutes.

Green Rice Casserole

2 cups cooked brown rice	1 cup chopped parsley
2 cups cheddar cheese, grated	1 small onion, chopped
	⅓ cup butter, melted
2 cups milk	2 eggs, well beaten

Mix all ingredients together. Bake at 350° for 45 minutes.

You will notice the addition of instant or nonfat powdered milk to some of these recipes. Powdered milk is measured the same as other dry ingredients, but never sifted. It may be added to either the dry or liquid ingredients in a recipe. Noninstant powdered milk is 50 percent higher in protein than instant. Noninstant would be found in health food stores.

General rules for using powdered milk are as follows: Ground meats, fish or chicken—use ½ to ¾ cups powdered milk to each pound of meat. Cooked cereal—mix equal amounts of powdered milk and cereal before cooking, then cook as directed on cereal package. Mashed vegetables such as potatoes, squash, sweet potatoes, rutabagas and turnips— add ⅓ cup powdered milk to each 2 cups of mashed vegetable, use cooking water to give the right consistency and season with butter, salt and pepper. Sauces, gravies, soups, custards—add 4 Tbsps. powdered milk to each cup of fluid milk or ½ cup powdered milk to each cup of water or broth in recipe.

Baked Custard

3 cups fresh milk
¼ cup powdered nonfat milk
½ cup honey

¼ tsp. salt
4 eggs
1 tsp. vanilla
Nutmeg

Preheat oven to 325°. Mix powdered milk, honey, and salt with fresh milk and scald. Add to beaten eggs, stirring well. Add vanilla. Pour into custard cups. Sprinkle with nutmeg. Bake 45 minutes in pan of hot water.

Yogurt Orange Drink

2 cups plain yogurt
1 cup orange juice

2 Tbsps. honey

Combine all ingredients and mix well using blender or egg beater. Other fruit juices may be used in place of orange juice.

Yogurt Dressing

1 cup plain yogurt
1 cup mayonnaise or salad dressing

1 Tbsp. vinegar or lemon juice

Mix with egg beater or electric mixer. Do not use blender.

Cottage Cheese Sherbet

1½ cups cottage cheese
1 Tbsp. lemon juice
1 tsp. grated lemon peel

½ cup honey
1½ cups yogurt

Blend all ingredients in blender until smooth. Turn into ice-cube tray of refrigerator. Stir twice while freezing.

Sesame Seed Squares

½ cup honey
½ cup peanut butter
1 cup powdered nonfat
   milk

½ cup unsweetened coconut
1 cup sesame seeds

Heat honey and peanut butter slightly over very low heat for ease of mixing. Add powdered milk, coconut and sesame seeds. Mix well and pat into oiled 9″ square pan. Place in refrigerator to set. Cut in squares. (Approximately 60 calories per square with 4 grams of good-quality protein per square. Absolutely delicious!)

Peanut Butter Candy

1 cup pure old-fashioned
   crunchy peanut butter

1 cup honey
2 cups powdered milk

Combine all ingredients thoroughly. Shape into one-inch balls and roll in coconut or crushed nuts.

Carobnog

3 tsps. carob powder
1 Tbsp. honey
1 beaten egg

2 cups milk
¼ tsp. vanilla
½ cup heavy cream, whipped

Combine carob, honey, and beaten egg and beat or blend. Add milk and vanilla and blend again. Top each serving with a dollop of whipped cream. Serves eight.

You will find recipes in other sections that also contain milk. It is not too difficult to see to it that family members receive an adequate intake of milk when you realize how many recipes call for it.

Proteins: Meat, Fish, Legumes, Eggs

When planning meals, we usually plan them around the meat or protein dish. (This will include not only meat but also fish, poultry, eggs, dried beans and peas.)

Meat. Liver is the most nutritious form of meat, as it is the storage organ of the animal. We will start with liver recipes. Many people object to the somewhat bitter taste of liver, but this can be largely alleviated by marinating the liver for several minutes in lemon juice or vinegar.

Broiled Liver

1 pound sliced beef or   ¼ cup lemon juice
  calves' liver   2 Tbsps. vegetable oil

Rinse liver in running water. Pat dry with paper towels. Soak liver in lemon juice 15 minutes. Drain and brush liver with oil. Broil on each side long enough for liver to heat through and change color. Season with salt and pepper.

Sautéed Liver and Onions

1 pound lamb or calves'   ½ cup wheat germ
  liver   2 Tbsps. dry milk
¼ cup vinegar   ½ tsp. salt
3 onions, chopped   ¼ tsp. marjoram
3 Tbsps. vegetable oil

Rinse liver in running water. Pat dry with paper towels. Soak liver in vinegar 15 minutes. Drain. Heat oil, sauté onions 5 minutes. Combine wheat germ, dry milk, salt, and marjoram, and dip liver in mixture. Sauté 5 minutes on each side. Serve hot.

Liver-and-Beef Loaf

1 pound ground beef   2 onions, chopped
½ pound ground liver   ¼ cup celery and tops,
1 cup wheat germ   chopped
1 egg   1 tsp. salt

Preheat oven to 350°. Mix all ingredients. Bake in oiled loaf pan for one hour.

Chopped Beef Curry

You can stretch a pound of chopped beef to serve four generously by making it into an unusual and flavorful curry. It is good to look at and good to eat. Serve on hot, fluffy, brown rice and add a vegetable. Serve cole slaw instead of salad, and for dessert try fruit-flavor gelatin with fresh fruit folded in.

1 tart apple, peeled, cored, chopped	1 tsp. salt
2 medium onions, finely chopped	½ cup diced celery
1 garlic clove, minced	⅓ cup raisins
1 lb. lean ground beef	¼ cup flaked coconut
1 Tbsp. curry powder (to taste)	1 can (10½ oz.) beef gravy (or make your own)
	1 can (8 oz.) tomato sauce

Sauté apple, onions, and garlic in oil for 5 minutes. Add beef, break up with fork; brown slowly. Sprinkle with curry powder and salt. Add remaining ingredients; mix well. Simmer, covered, about 40 minutes (check). Serve on rice with any desired curry accompaniments in addition to those mentioned— chutney, peanuts, diced cucumber. Makes 4 generous servings.

Escalopes of Veal

6 veal slices, ½″ thick	½ tsp. seasoned salt
⅓ cup butter	2 Tbsps. chopped parsley
1 cup stock (bouillon cube and hot water)	2 Tbsps. chopped onion
¼ tsp. garlic powder	Salt and pepper to taste

Pound veal gently with edge of saucer until thin. Melt butter. Sauté veal for 3 minutes on each side, until brown. Add other ingredients. Cover, simmer on low flame 20 minutes. Serve with *Tomato Sauce Provençale*.

Tomato Sauce Provençale

8 large tomatoes	1 clove garlic
1 large onion, thinly	1 Tbsp. butter
sliced	½ tsp. salt
¼ tsp. thyme	¼ tsp. pepper
1 bay leaf	1 Tbsp. unbleached flour

Simmer all ingredients except flour for 20 minutes. Make paste of flour and a few Tbsps. water and add to other ingredients. Simmer slowly, stirring, for a few minutes until thickened.

Chili With Beans

¼ cup vegetable oil	1 Tbsp. chili powder
½ cup onion, chopped	1 cup tomato puree
½ cup green pepper,	2 tsps. salt
chopped	2 cups cooked pinto or
1 pound ground beef	kidney beans

Sauté onions and green peppers until tender. Add meat and sauté until it loses red color. Add seasonings, tomato puree, and beans. Simmer over low heat for one hour. (*Note*: Adjust amount of chili powder for individual taste.)

Poultry. An excellent source of protein, chicken and other poultry products adapt easily to family and company-style recipes. Poultry is generally low in fat, nutritious, and economical.

Oven-Fried Chicken

1 cut-up frying chicken	1 tsp. salt
½ cup evaporated milk	⅛ tsp. pepper
½ cup whole-wheat flour	¼ cup oil
½ cup wheat germ	

Preheat oven to 350°. Combine flour, wheat germ, salt, and pepper. Dip pieces of chicken in milk, then roll in mixture. Bake in oiled shallow baking pan uncovered for 1 hour.

Many basic recipes are easily adapted for party times. Double or triple amounts given, depending on the size of the group. The next two chicken recipes are well-suited for such occasions. The chicken salad is very festive and attractive. If you have an extra punch bowl, make it for a large Christmas gathering and expect everyone to ask for the recipe.

Chicken Salad

1 large stewing chicken (or equivalent in breasts)
1 8-oz. package shell macaroni
1 cup salad dressing (or more)
1 bunch celery, diced
2 pkgs. frozen peas, cooked, drained, and cooled

1 large bottle stuffed olives, sliced
10 hard-cooked eggs, cut in pieces
1 No. 2 can pineapple chunks, drained
1 large package cashew nuts
2 heads lettuce (torn in bite-size pieces. Save outer leaves)

Stew chicken until tender (or sauté breasts). Prepare macaroni according to package directions. Drain and cool. Marinate bite-sized pieces of cooled chicken and macaroni several hours in 1 cup salad dressing. Gently combine with rest of ingredients, adding more salad dressing if needed. Add nuts just before serving in large attractive bowl lined with outer leaves of lettuce.

Scalloped Chicken Casserole

1 large stewing chicken (or 4–6 chicken breasts)

If using stewing chicken, gently simmer in 4 cups water with 1 tsp. salt. Or brown breasts in oil until tender. When cooled, separate meat from bones and cut in bite-size pieces. Set aside.

Stuffing
1 onion, chopped
½ cup melted butter
2 stalks celery, chopped

4 cups seasoned stuffing mix
½ cup (about) evaporated milk

Sauté onion in butter, add celery. Pour over stuffing mix. Moisten with evaporated milk.

Sauce

½ cup melted butter (add to   3 cups chicken broth
pan drippings from breasts).   (canned, or broth from
4 Tbsps. unbleached flour   stewing chicken)

Combine all ingredients and cook, stirring, over low heat until thickened.

Assemble Casserole: Place layer of stuffing in bottom of oiled 3-quart casserole. Next add a layer of chicken, then another layer of stuffing. Pour some sauce over. Alternate this layering, ending with stuffing. Sprinkle with ½ cup (or more) sliced almonds. Bake at 350° for 35 minutes or until bubbly.

Poulet de Broccoli

2⅔ cups cooked chicken breast   ½ tsp. curry powder
and thigh, in chunks   1¼ cups sharp cheddar
2 pkgs. frozen broccoli or   cheese, grated
fresh equivalent   1¼ cups bread crumbs
2 cans cream of chicken soup   2 Tbsps. melted butter
1 tsp. lemon juice

Barely cook broccoli. (Slash stems for more even cooking.) Put in buttered casserole. Add layer of chicken. Cover with mixture of soup, lemon juice, curry powder. Top with mixture of crumbs, cheese, butter. Bake at 350° for 30 minutes or until bubbly. Serves 8. Use cooked turkey for variation.

Hot Turkey Salad

2 cups cooked diced turkey   ½ tsp. salt
2 cups chopped celery   2 tsps. grated onion
½ cup chopped almonds   ¾ cup grated cheese
1 cup mayonnaise   1 cup bread crumbs
2 Tbsps. lemon juice

Mix turkey, celery, and almonds. Blend mayonnaise, lemon juice, salt, and onion. Mix lightly with the turkey mixture. Spoon into oiled 9″ square pan. Sprinkle grated cheese and crumbs on top. Bake at 450° for 10 minutes. Serve hot. Serves 6–8. Garnish with parsley. Variation: cooked chicken or tuna.

Lemon-Honey Chicken

8 pieces of chicken
2 Tbsps. butter, melted
⅓ cup whole-wheat flour
1 tsp. salt
¼ tsp. pepper
¼ cup lemon juice
⅓ cup honey
1 Tbsp. soy souce

Brush chicken with melted butter; then coat with flour seasoned with salt and pepper. Put, skin side up, in lightly oiled baking dish. Pour other ingredients over (well-mixed). Bake at 350° for 1 hour or until done.

Coconut-Curry Chicken

⅓ cup frozen orange-juice
   concentrate, thawed
1 tsp. salt
1 egg, slightly beaten
1 3-pound frying chicken,
   cut up
½ cup wheat germ
½ cup crushed cornflakes
½ cup shredded coconut
1 tsp. curry powder
¼ cup butter, melted
Orange slices

Mix first 3 ingredients. Add chicken, marinate 15 minutes. Mix next 4 ingredients. Coat chicken with mixture, pressing it on. Put on lightly oiled foil-lined pan and drizzle with butter combined with reserved marinade. Cover pan with foil and bake at 350° for 30 minutes. Uncover and bake 30 to 40 minutes longer or until well browned. Serve on platter with garnish of fresh oranges sliced. Serves 4–6.

Fish. Food from the sea is an excellent source of protein, especially since it is lower in fat content than meat.

Tuna and Rice

1¼ cups cooked brown rice
½ can cream of mushroom
   soup
⅓ cup evaporated milk
1 7-ounce can tuna fish

½ cup shredded cheddar
   cheese
¼ cup onion, chopped
¼ cup chopped pimento or
   green pepper

Preheat oven to 350°. Combine all ingredients and mix well. Put in oiled baking dish. Bake 30 minutes or until bubbly. Serves 4.

Baked Herbed Fish

2 pounds fresh fish fillets
   (or frozen, slightly thawed)
½ cup butter
1 onion, chopped
½ cup milk

½ tsp. salt
⅛ tsp. pepper
¼ tsp. marjoram
¼ tsp. tarragon
1 Tbsp. minced parsley

Heat oven to 350°. Place fillets in oiled baking dish. Dot with butter and sprinkle with chopped onion and seasonings. Pour over the milk. Bake about 20 minutes or until fish flakes with a fork. Serves 4–6.

Seafood Au Gratin

½ lb. cooked lobster
½ lb. cooked shrimp
2 slices American cheese

½ cup milk
Salt and pepper to taste
½ tsp. paprika

Melt cheese with milk in double boiler. Combine all ingredients and put in oiled casserole. Top with buttered crumbs. Bake at 350° for about 20 minutes or until bubbly. Serves 4.

Crabmeat Puffs

6 slices bread, crusts removed
   (whole wheat preferred)
3 slices American cheese
1 cup crabmeat

2 eggs
1 cup milk
½ tsp. salt
Pepper to taste

Lay 3 bread slices across bottom of oiled baking dish. Cover with cheese, then crabmeat. Top with remaining bread. Beat eggs with milk and seasonings. Pour over other ingredients. Chill for 2 hours. Bake at 350° for 30 minutes or until puffy. Serve at once.

Flounder Rolls With Carrot Stuffing

2 lbs. flounder fillets (or sole), fresh or frozen
1 tsp. salt
⅛ tsp. white pepper
2 cups finely shredded carrot
¼ cup finely chopped onion
¼ cup butter
2 Tbsps. chopped parsley
1 can cream of celery soup
1 can (4 oz.) sliced, drained mushrooms
2 Tbsps. lemon juice

Sprinkle fillets with salt and pepper. Sauté carrot and onion in butter until onion is tender but not brown. Stir in parsley. Spread an equal amount of carrot mixture over each fillet. Roll up and secure with skewers or wooden picks. Combine soup, mushrooms, and lemon juice. Pour into shallow 1½-quart baking dish. Arrange rolls in soup mixture. Bake at 350° about 30 minutes or until fish flakes easily with a fork. Spoon sauce over rolls several times during baking. Serves 6–8.

Beans. Give your purse and your heart a break—serve beans! The American Heart Association has advised Americans that they should cut their meat consumption by one-third. We can do this by cashing in on the bean bonanza. Beans are also a good food for weight watchers, and don't let anyone tell you otherwise! A half-cup of cooked white or red beans is only 118 calories (that is 3.5 ounces—and steak would give you 465 calories). Beans contain less than 2 percent fat, and they are the kinds you need—linoleic and linolenic fatty acids. Search out recipes and watch for ways to serve and use beans. In particular, experiment with soybeans, for they are supernutritious and so versatile. You will also want to use peas and lentils. The basic recipe given is generally a family favorite.

Split Pea Soup

4 cups water	1 tsp. salt
1 cup split peas	⅛ tsp. pepper
(or dried beans)	1 carrot, diced
1 onion, chopped	1 bay leaf (optional)

Wash peas. Bring water to a boil and add split peas slowly. Cook at a simmer until peas are tender. Watch carefully, and stir as needed to prevent sticking. More water may be needed. Add rest of ingredients and simmer another 30 minutes. You may wish to press the soup through a sieve before serving. (Add leftover diced ham, if desired.)

Eggs. What turns a simple egg into something special? Practice, use a well-seasoned skillet, and you can turn out a magnificent omelet every time. We will give you the basic omelet recipe, and once you have mastered the technique, you can add elegantly simple fillings, such as sautéed mushrooms, green peppers, minced onion, spinach—you will be limited only by your imagination. Any vegetable (seasoned to your liking with herbs and/or spices) can be adapted as an omelet filling. Even fruits (and jams) can be used for a simple luncheon-type omelet.

Basic Omelet (One Serving)

2 eggs	¼ tsp. salt
1 Tbsp. water	1 Tbsp. butter

Place eggs, water, and salt in bowl. Beat with a fork until blended. Do not overbeat. Heat butter in a 6- to 8-inch skillet until it sizzles but does not brown. Tilt pan until bottom is coated. Pour in egg mixture and stir briskly with flat bottom of fork, at the same time shaking the pan to prevent sticking. Let cook further, without stirring, over medium heat, lifting edges to let uncooked egg run underneath. When bottom is slightly brown and top is moist but not runny, add filling. Remove pan from heat, tilt slightly and roll up or fold omelet with fork. Tip onto heated serving plate.

Omelet Fillings (Single Serving)

4 Tbsps. sliced and lightly sautéed mushrooms
3 Tbsps. finely chopped and lightly sautéed shallots
2 Tbsps. finely chopped mixed herbs—parsley, chives, chervil, tarragon
4 Tbsps. chopped and sautéed green pepper
¼ cup shredded American cheese
½ cup diced avocado
¼ cup hot cooked spinach

Hard-Boiled Eggs

For perfect hard-boiled eggs every time: put eggs in a pan large enough so eggs don't touch each other. Add one cup of water per egg. Add salt to water. Now cover. Bring to a full rolling boil and then turn burner off. For hard-cooked eggs (as for a salad), leave in pan *without removing lid* for 15–18 minutes. (For soft-cooked eggs leave 1–2 minutes.) Now pour off water and add cold water. Drain again. Let cool. The eggs will be just right.

Chileo Rellano

3 eggs
1 block grated Jack cheese
1 block grated cheddar cheese

1 large can evaporated milk
2 Tbsps. unbleached flour
1 7-oz. can green chilies

Remove chili seeds. Lay in 9″ x 14″ baking dish. Layer cheese on chilies. Blend milk with eggs and flour. Pour over. Bake at 350° for 40 minutes.

Cheese Puff (Elegant for parties!)

9 slices whole wheat bread
Butter
1 lb. grated cheese
6 eggs

1 quart milk
1 tsp. salt
1 tsp. dry mustard

Preheat oven to 350°. Remove crusts from bread (save and use later, toasted, for salad). Butter bread. Oil a 9″ x 14″ baking dish. Lay slices of bread across bottom of dish. Add grated cheese and continue with layers of bread and cheese. Beat eggs with salt, mustard, and milk. Pour over layers in casserole. Let stand in refrigerator overnight. Bake next day for one hour. Serve immediately so puff won't fall.

Vegetable and Fruit Group

Vegetables should be cooked in as little water as possible, and in as short a time as possible in order to preserve valuable nutrients. The water in which vegetables are cooked should never be thrown away and can be used to advantage in sauces, soups, and stews.

Fruits should be eaten fresh and raw as much as possible. If canned or frozen at home, use no sugar or a very light syrup.

Salads, using combinations of raw or cooked vegetables and/or fruits, are excellent ways to add food from this group to the daily menu plan.

Sautéed Carrots

6 to 8 carrots	1 Tbsp. water
2 Tbsps. oil	1 tsp. salt

Dice or slice carrots. Put all ingredients in heavy pan, cover, heat quickly, and reduce temperature. Stir occasionally. Cook 10 to 15 minutes. Other root vegetables such as turnips, rutabagas, parsnips, or beets may be cooked in the same way.

Vegetables Cooked in Milk

1 or 2 pounds of any vegetable	1 or 2 Tbsps. butter
Milk	½ tsp. salt
	⅛ tsp. pepper

Prepare vegetable by dicing, slicing, or shredding. Add enough hot milk to barely cover. Simmer on low heat about 10 minutes or until tender. Add butter, salt, and pepper.

Broiled Eggplant

1 large eggplant	1 tsp. salt
¼ cup evaporated milk	2 Tbsps. oil
½ cup wheat germ	

Slice unpeeled eggplant. Dip slices in milk, then in wheat germ mixed with salt. Place on oiled broiler pan. Broil about 3 or 4 inches from heat until brown on one side, turn and brown other side.

Summer Squash or Zucchini with Tomatoes and Cheese

3 cups summer squash or zucchini	1 tsp. salt
1 onion chopped	½ cup diced cheddar cheese
2 Tbsps. vegetable oil	1 cup canned tomatoes

Cut squash into small pieces. Brown squash and onion in oil; cover and simmer on low heat 10 minutes. Add salt, cheese, and tomatoes. Heat until cheese melts.

Baked Tomatoes

3 large tomatoes	½ tsp. basil
¼ cup onion, chopped	½ tsp. salt
¼ cup parsley, chopped	½ cup shredded cheese
½ cup wheat germ	

Preheat oven to 350°. Cut tomatoes in half and place in oiled baking dish. Mix rest of ingredients together and spread over tomatoes. Bake in 350° oven for 8 to 10 minutes.

Steamed Beets and Beet Tops

8 to 10 tiny fresh beets with tops	1 tsp. salt
	2 Tbsps. vinegar

Wash beets and tops and cook in covered pan with enough water to cover them. Simmer slowly 10 to 15 minutes. Add salt and vinegar.

Broccoli or Brussels Sprouts With Mushroom Sauce

1 lb. broccoli or Brussels   ½ cup evaporated milk
 sprouts   1 tsp. salt
1 can cream of mushroom
 soup

Mix soup with milk and heat to simmering. Add the cleaned and cut-up broccoli or the whole Brussels sprouts. Simmer until tender, about 10 –12 minutes.

Cauliflower With Cheese Sauce

1 head cauliflower   1 cup diced cheddar
2 cups milk   cheese
2 Tbsps. unbleached flour   1 tsp. salt

Heat the milk to simmering, add cauliflower, broken into flowerets. Simmer over low heat, 10–15 minutes. Remove cauliflower. Make paste of flour and a few Tbsps. cold milk. Add to balance of milk used to cook cauliflower. Cook, stirring, until thickened. Add cheese and salt; stir until melted. Pour over reserved cauliflower to serve.

Roasted Corn on the Cob

6 ears fresh corn,   2 Tbsps. fortified butter
 unhusked   Salt and pepper to taste

Preheat oven to 400°. Remove outer husks of corn, leaving 1 or 2 layers to prevent drying out. Pull these back and spread with soft butter, salt, pepper. Replace husks and roast in hot oven for 10–12 minutes.

Cantaloupe Cup

Cantaloupes   Mixed fruits

Cut cantaloupes in half. Flute edges if desired. Cut out part of pulp and dice it. Fill center with diced cantaloupe and other fruits such as diced pineapple, sliced peaches or apricots, sweet pitted cherries, strawberries, raspberries. Chill well.

Filled Pineapple Halves

1 large pineapple
2 cups strawberries

¼ cup honey

Cut pineapple in half lengthwise. Scoop out pulp and dice it. Mix with strawberries and honey. Fill pineapple halves.

Minted Cantaloupe Medley

¾ cup honey
2 Tbsps. lime juice
1 tsp. chopped fresh mint
½ tsp. anise seed

Dash salt
5 cups cantaloupe slices
3 cups fresh peach slices
2 cups blueberries

Combine honey and lime juice, mint, anise, salt. Simmer all for 2 minutes. Cover and steep 10 minutes. Cool and chill. Place fruit in large bowl and strain syrup over fruit to remove anise. Cover and chill 2 hours or until ready to serve (same day). Makes 10 servings. Other fruits may be substituted.

Apple Salad With Pineapple

2 medium Golden Delicious
   apples (cored and cut in
   large dice)
1 14-oz. can pineapple
   tidbits

2 Tbsps. chopped dill
   pickle
¼ cup mayonnaise
⅛ tsp. salt

Mix all together and serve on lettuce cup.

Apple Salad With Grapes

2 medium red apples (cored
   and cut in large dice)
1 cup halved, seeded grapes
¼ cup toasted slivered
   almonds

¼ cup sour cream
1 tsp. lemon juice
1 Tbsp. honey
¼ tsp. salt
⅛ tsp. dry mustard

Mix all together and serve on lettuce cup.

Tossed Salad

The bases of tossed salads are the various kinds of lettuce. Other raw vegetables may be added, such as tomatoes, radishes, green onions, cucumbers, celery, and even other tender greens such as spinach, chard, and so on.

1 head lettuce	2 tomatoes
1 bunch of radishes	¼ tsp. each of seasoned
1 bunch of green onions	salt and garlic salt
1 cucumber	⅓ cup French dressing

Break up lettuce into bite-size pieces in large salad bowl. Add sliced radishes, onions, cucumbers, and quartered tomatoes. Sprinkle with salts. Just before serving toss well but lightly with French dressing. See end of salad section for dressing recipes.

Wilted Spinach Salad Supreme

4 slices crisp bacon, drained	1 lb. raw spinach
1 Tbsp. bacon drippings	2 hard-cooked eggs, peeled and sliced
4 Tbsps. fine-grade olive oil	Sweet onion rings
3 Tbsps. wine vinegar	

Wash spinach and drain well. Mix bacon drippings, olive oil, and vinegar in glass jar. Sprinkle this over greens, eggs, onion rings, crumbled bacon. Season with salt and pepper to taste.

Avocado Salad

2 medium avocados	¼ tsp. chili powder
2 Tbsps. lemon juice	⅛ tsp. oregano
2 tsps. mayonnaise	Salt, pepper
2 Tbsps. diced mushrooms	Dash hot pepper sauce
2 Tbsps. diced peeled tomatoes	

Serve on lettuce with carrot sticks, green pepper rings and wedges of tomatoes. 4 servings.

Avocado Cashew Salad

1 3-oz. pkg. lime gelatin
1⅔ cups hot water
2 Tbsps. lime or lemon
  juice

1 large avocado, mashed
⅓ lb. cashew nuts,
  chopped

Dissolve gelatin in hot water. Add lime juice. Chill until beginning to thicken. Fold in avocado and nuts. Chill until firm. Serve on greens. 6 servings.

Vegetable Salad

Lettuce
1 cup diced cooked beets
½ cup cooked green beans
1 hard-cooked egg

½ cup celery, sliced diagonally
¼ cup diced cheese
½ tsp. garlic salt
¼ cup mayonnaise

Arrange lettuce leaves on salad plates. Combine all other ingredients except mayonnaise and mix lightly. Just before serving add mayonnaise and put on lettuce cups.

Cole Slaw

1 head cabbage, finely
  shredded
1 cup yogurt

¼ cup vinegar
2 Tbsps. honey
1 tsp. salt

Combine yogurt, vinegar, honey, and salt. Mix well. Add to cabbage. Diced green pepper, shredded carrots, celery, or diced cucumber may be added.

Carrot Salad

2 lbs. cooked carrots
  (do not overcook)

1 medium bell pepper, sliced
1 medium onion, sliced

Dressing

1 can tomato soup
1½ tsps. vegetable oil
¾ cup honey

¾ cup cider vinegar
1 tsp. dry mustard (or prepared)
Salt and pepper

Whip the dressing ingredients together. Pour over drained carrots and other vegetables. Store in refrigerator at least 8–12 hours before serving. Will keep well in refrigerator for some time.

Avocado Party Dip

1 ripe avocado	Juice of ½ lemon
½ cup mayonnaise	Few drops hot pepper
½ tsp. salt	sauce
1 slice onion	

Peel avocado and cut into pieces. Place in blender with remaining ingredients. Blend until smooth. Allow to stand in refrigerator 1 hour. Garnish with sliced stuffed olives. Makes about ¾ cup.

Sliced Tomatoes With Herb Dressing

Slice beefsteak tomatoes about ¼″ thick. Overlap slices in shallow bowl, tucking onion slices in between. Sprinkle with freshly ground black pepper. Drizzle *Basil Dressing* over all: Combine in blender—¼ cup olive oil, 2 Tbsps. red wine vinegar (garlic flavored), ½ tsp. salt, ½ tsp. honey, ¼ cup fresh basil leaves (or 1 Tbsp. dried whole basil).

Cottage Cheese Party Dip

1 cup cottage cheese	½ cup chives
1 Tbsp. lemon juice	½ tsp. seasoned salt
½ tsp. garlic powder	½ tsp. paprika

Mix all ingredients together and set out in bowl surrounded by raw vegetables for dipping.

Herb Dressing

1 cup sour cream	½ tsp. salt
1 cup mayonnaise	⅛ tsp. pepper
1 small onion, chopped	¼ tsp. paprika
2 Tbsps. lemon juice	⅛ tsp. curry powder

½ tsp. dried herbs (thyme,   1 tsp. caraway seeds
   rosemary, basil   1 clove garlic, minced
½ tsp. Worcestershire sauce   1 tsp. chopped parsley

Blend all ingredients. Chill 24 hours before serving.

French Dressing

¾ cup oil   ¼ tsp. garlic salt
¼ cup vinegar   ⅛ tsp. pepper
2 tsps. honey   ½ tsp. paprika
1 tsp. salt

Combine all ingredients in a jar. Shake until well blended. (Or put ingredients in blender and whirl.) Store in refrigerator and shake well before using.

Tomato French Dressing

1 cup tomato catsup   1 tsp. salt
¾ cup vegetable oil   1 tsp. dry mustard
½ cup cider vinegar   1 tsp. celery seed
1 medium onion, chopped 1 tsp. caraway seed
1 clove garlic, minced   ½ tsp. ground rosemary
⅓ cup honey

Place all ingredients in blender and mix well. Store in refrigerator and shake well before using.

Yogurt-Honey Dressing

1 cup yogurt   2 Tbsps. honey
1 Tbsp. lemon juice   ⅛ tsp. mace

Combine all ingredients and mix well. Store in refrigerator.

Fruit Juice Yogurt Dressing

1 cup yogurt   2 Tbsps. orange juice
1 Tbsp. honey   2 Tbsps. pineapple juice

Combine all ingredients and mix well. Serve with fruit salads.

Yogurt-Blue Cheese Dressing

1 cup yogurt   1 Tbsp. chives
½ cup blue cheese

Crumble blue cheese. Mix with yogurt and chives. Good on tossed salads.

Breads and Cereals

We recommend the use of whole grains only, whether in flour, bread, or breakfast cereals.

Crunchy Granola

4 cups rolled oats   ½ cup unprocessed
1½ cups shredded unsweetened   bran flakes
   coconut   1 cup ground roasted
1 cup wheat germ   soybeans
1 cup chopped nuts   ½ cup oil
1 cup hulled sunflower seeds   ½ cup honey
½ cup sesame seeds   1 tsp. vanilla

Heat oven to 325°. Mix together all of the dry ingredients thoroughly. Combine oil, honey, and vanilla. Heat (do not boil). Add the honey-oil mixture to the dry ingredients. Spread the mixture on oiled cookie sheets. Bake about 15 minutes until light brown, turning occasionally. Serve as a breakfast cereal with milk, or may be eaten dry as a snack.

Bible Bread

1 pkg. dry yeast   2 Tbsps. oil
1 Tbsp. honey   1 tsp. salt
1¼ cups lukewarm water   3½ cups whole wheat
   or milk   flour

Dissolve yeast and honey in lukewarm liquid. Add oil, salt, and flour. Mix well and knead. Cut dough into 8 pieces, and shape into rounds. Roll out until about 5″ across and ¼″ thick. Place on lightly oiled cookie sheets. Cover with clean towel and let rise in warm place until ½″ to ¾″ thick. Bake at 450° for 8–10 minutes. This is similar to the bread which Jesus ate.

American Indian Fry Bread

1 cup unsifted whole wheat flour	2 Tbsps. dry milk
½ cup enriched cornmeal	½ cup warm water
1 tsp. baking powder	½ cup vegetable oil (for frying)
1 tsp. salt	1 tsp. baking powder

Mix dry ingredients. Stir in warm water. Knead 5 minutes. Let stand one-half hour. Take a piece the size of large lemon and roll flat to about 6″ diameter. Fry one at a time in hot oil.

Nature's Way
Whole-Wheat Bread

1½ cups warm milk	½ Tbsp. salt
¼ cup honey	3 to 4 cups whole wheat flour
2 pkgs. dry yeast	
¼ cup vegetable oil	

Combine milk, honey, and yeast. Let set 5 minutes. Add oil, salt, and half of flour. Beat thoroughly. Add rest of flour and knead. Let rise in warm place until double in size. Punch down, knead, and let rise again. Punch down and form into loaves and place in well-greased loaf pans. Let rise again until double. Bake in preheated oven at 400° for 40 to 50 minutes or until done.

Wheat-Germ Rolls

1 cup warm milk	1 egg
¼ cup honey	½ cup wheat germ
2 pkgs. dry yeast	2 tsps. salt
⅓ cup oil	2½ cups whole wheat flour

Combine milk, honey, and yeast, and let set 5 minutes. Add rest of ingredients, mix well, and knead. Let rise in warm place until double. Punch down and form into rolls. Let rise again. Bake in preheated oven at 375° for 20 to 25 minutes.

Pancakes

1 cup whole wheat flour	1 tsp. baking soda
½ cup wheat germ	2 eggs
½ cup cornmeal	2 Tbsps. vegetable oil
1 tsp. salt	1½ cups yogurt

Combine dry ingredients. Beat together the eggs, oil, and yogurt. Add to dry mixture. Bake on hot griddle.

Bran Muffins

1½ cups whole wheat flour	1 cup milk
3 tsps. baking powder	⅓ cup vegetable oil
1 tsp. salt	1 egg
⅓ cup honey or molasses	½ cup raisins or nuts
1½ cups bran buds	(optional)

Heat oven to 400°. Combine flour, baking powder, salt. Add bran buds to milk and let set for 2 minutes. Add egg, oil, and honey to bran mixture. Stir in dry ingredients, mixing only until combined. Bake about 20 to 25 minutes in paper-lined muffin cups.

Toasted Wheat Germ

3 cups fresh wheat germ	⅓ cup honey

Preheat oven to 300°. Mix wheat germ and honey and spread on cookie sheet. Bake for 10 minutes, turning occasionally. May be served as a cold cereal with milk, or as a topping for desserts.

Four-Week Bran Muffins

4 cups Kellogg's All Bran	4 eggs beaten
2 cups Nabisco 100% Bran	1 quart buttermilk
1¾ cups boiling water	5 cups whole wheat or
1 cup raisins	unbleached flour
1 cup fortified butter	5 tsps. baking soda
(with vegetable oil)	1 tsp. salt
2 cups honey	

Mix bran products, raisins, and water together and set aside to cool. Sift dry ingredients together. Combine all ingredients and store in airtight container in refrigerator. Do not stir when ready to use—spoon into paper-lined muffin cups. Bake at 375° for 20 to 25 minutes. Handy to have on hand for breakfast or any time!

Cakes. We do not recommend the use of commercial cake mixes, as they are made from refined, nonenriched flour, saturated fats, and sugar. The only real nutrition in them is found in the two eggs we add. Delicious cakes can be made in other ways.

Scripture Cake

¾ cup fortified butter	Genesis 18:8
1½ cups brown or raw sugar	Jeremiah 6:20
5 eggs	Luke 11:12
3 cups whole wheat flour	Leviticus 24:5
¾ tsp. salt	2 Kings 2:20
3 tsps. baking powder	Amos 4:5
1 tsp. cinnamon	Exodus 30:23
¼ tsp. each cloves, allspice, and nutmeg	2 Chronicles 9:9
½ cup milk	Judges 4:19
½ cup chopped walnuts	Genesis 43:11
½ cup dried figs or dates, cut up	Jeremiah 24:5
½ cup raisins	2 Samuel 16:1

Heat oven to 350°. Cream butter, sugar, and eggs thoroughly. Combine all dry ingredients and add alternately to creamed mixture with the milk. Stir in nuts and fruits. Bake in two oiled cake pans for about 30 to 40 minutes.

Unbaked Fruit Cake

2 cups pitted dates	2 cups walnuts, chopped
2 cups pitted prunes	2 cups shredded coconut
2 cups seedless raisins	1 cup honey

Grind all ingredients and mix thoroughly with honey. Press firmly into oiled loaf pans. Refrigerate for one day or longer. Will keep in refrigerator for two or three weeks.

Baked Fruit Cake

2 cups whole-wheat pastry
   flour
3 tsps. baking powder
½ cup apple cider
½ cup vegetable oil

1 cup honey
1 cup applesauce
1 cup nuts, chopped
1 cup dates, chopped
1 cup seedless raisins

Heat oven to 350°. Combine cider, honey, oil, and applesauce. Add flour and baking powder and mix well. Add nuts and fruits. Bake for about 1 hour in oiled pan. Allow cake to ripen for a day or two before cutting.

Baked Cheesecake

1½ cups graham cracker
   crumbs
⅓ cup melted butter
2 eggs
¾ cup honey

2 cups cottage cheese
¼ cup powdered milk
2 tsps. vanilla
1 tsp. almond extract

Heat oven to 300°. Combine crumbs and butter. (Crush crackers in plastic bag by rolling fine.) Press into bottom and sides of pie pan. Mix all other ingredients and beat until smooth. Pour into crust. Set on jar lids in a pan of boiling water and bake for 30 minutes. Top with thickened cherries, strawberries or other fruit.

Oatmeal Cookies

3 cups rolled oats
1½ cups wheat germ
1 cup whole wheat flour
2 tsps. baking powder
1 tsp. salt
¾ cup vegetable oil

1 cup sorghum or molasses
2 eggs
2 tsps. vanilla
1 cup raisins and/or chopped
   nuts

Heat oven to 350°. Combine all dry ingredients. Mix together all wet ingredients and combine the two mixtures. Add raisins and/or nuts. Drop by teaspoons onto oiled cookie sheet. Bake 10 to 12 minutes.

Wheat-Germ Brownies

¼ cup vegetable oil
1 cup brown sugar or honey
2 eggs
1 tsp. vanilla
½ tsp. salt

1 cup wheat germ
¼ cup carob powder
½ cup powdered milk
1 tsp. baking powder
1 cup chopped nuts

Heat oven to 325°. Combine oil, sugar, eggs, vanilla. Beat well. Add dry ingredients and nuts. Spread in 8″ by 8″ oiled pan. Bake for 40 minutes.

Pie Crisp

2 cups whole wheat flour
1 tsp. salt

½ cup vegetable oil
¼ cup cold water

Heat oven to 400°. Combine flour and salt. Mix oil and water and cut into flour with pastry blender. Form into ball, divide, and roll out on floured board. Fit into pie pan. Bake for 10 to 15 minutes.

Gingerbread

⅓ cup vegetable oil
1 egg
1 cup molasses
½ cup yogurt
1 cup whole wheat flour
½ cup wheat germ

1 tsp. baking soda
¼ cup powdered milk
2 tsps. ginger
1 tsp. cinnamon
½ tsp. salt

Heat oven to 350°. Beat together oil, egg, and molasses. Mix dry ingredients thoroughly. Add to molasses mixture alternately with yogurt. Pour batter into square pan. Bake 40 to 45 minutes.

Bulgur. This is a whole-wheat product made by soaking in water, cooking, then drying. It may be left whole kernel, or ground coarse, medium, or fine. It goes by the commercial name of Ala or Bulghor. It keeps well because the particles are too hard for insects to bite into. Bulgur combined with meat, eggs, milk, or cheese makes a highly nutritious dish.

Crunchy Bulgur

2 cups bulgur   6 cups water   1 tsp. salt

Bring water to boil, add bulgur and salt. Cover pan, and cook over low heat about 20 minutes. It may be served as a breakfast cereal, or can be cooked in chicken or beef broth, and served in place of potatoes or rice to accompany meat.

Bulgur Meat Loaf

1 lb. ground beef   ¼ cup powdered milk
½ cup cooked bulgur   2 Tbsp. catsup
1 cup water   1 tsp. salt

Heat oven to 325°. Mix all ingredients. Place in oiled loaf pan. Bake for 45 minutes.

Meat Stew with Bulgur

1 lb. stew meat   ¼ tsp. pepper
2 Tbsps. oil   ¼ cup onions, diced
5 cups water   2 cups potatoes, diced
½ cup uncooked bulgur   1 cup carrots, diced
1½ tsps. salt   1 cup celery, diced

Brown meat in oil. Add water and simmer meat until tender—about 2 hours. Add bulgur, vegetables, and seasonings. Cook 20 minutes.

Bulgur Pilaf

1 envelope dried onion soup mix   1 cup diced chicken
1 cup uncooked bulgur   or meat
3 cups water

Add the soup mix and bulgur to water. Cover and simmer 20 minutes. Remove from heat and let stand 5 to 10 minutes. Add chicken or meat and heat.

Recommended Reading

Abrahamson, E. M., and Pezet, A. W. *Body, Mind & Sugar*. New York: Pyramid, 1951.

Albright, Nancy, ed. *The Rodale Cookbook*. Emmaus, Pa.: Rodale Press Inc., 1973.

Anderson, Lynn. *Rainbow Farm Cookbook*. New York: Harper and Row Publishers, Inc., 1973.

Bailey, Herbert. *Vitamin E: Your Key to a Healthy Heart*. New York: Arc Books, 1968.

Blaine, Tom R. *Goodbye Allergies*. Secaucus, N.J.: Citadel Press, 1968.

Blevin, Margo, and Ginder, Geri. *The Low Blood Sugar Cookbook*. New York: Doubleday and Company, Inc., 1973.

Braaten, Carl E., and Braaten, LaVonne. *The Living Temple: A Practical Theology of the Body and the Foods of the Earth*. New York: Harper and Row Publishers, Inc., 1976.

Brown, Edith, and Brown, Sam. *Cooking Creatively with Natural Foods*. New York: Ballatine Books, Inc., 1973.

Carson, Mary B., ed. *Womanly Art of Breastfeeding*, 2nd ed. Oak Park, Ill.: La Leche League, 1971.

Chen, Philip S. *Soybeans for Health and a Longer Life*. New Canaan, Conn.: Keats Publishing, 1974.

Cheraskin, Emanuel, et al. *Psycho-Dietetics: Food As the Key to Emotional Health*. New York: Stein and Day, 1974.

Cheraskin, E., et al. *Diet and Disease*. Emmaus, Pa.: Rodale Press, Inc., 1968.

Cheraskin, E., and Ringsdorf, W. M., Jr. *Predictive Medicine: A Study in Strategy*. Mountain View, Calif.: Pacific Press Publishing Association, 1973.

Clark, Linda. *Know Your Nutrition*. New Canaan, Conn.: Keats Publishing, Inc., 1973.

Clark, Linda. *Help Yourself to Health*. New York: Pyramid Publications, 1974.

Cleave, T. L. *Saccharine Disease: The Master Disease of Our Time*. New Canaan, Conn.: Keats Publishing, Inc., 1975.

Coca, Arthur F. *Pulse Test*. New York: Arc Books, 1968.

Cott, Allan. *Fasting: The Ultimate Diet*. New York: Bantam Books, 1975.

Crenshaw, Mary Ann. *The Natural Way to Super Beauty*. New York: Dell Publishing Co., Inc., 1975.

Cross, Jennifer. *The Supermarket Trap: The Consumer and the Food Industry*. Bloomington, Ind.: Indiana University Press, 1970.

Dankenbring, William E. *Your Keys to Radiant Health*. New Canaan, Conn.: Keats Publishing, Inc., 1974.

Davis, Adelle. *Let's Cook It Right,* rev. ed. New York: Harcourt Brace Jovanovich, 1962.

Davis, Adelle. *Let's Eat Right and Keep Fit.* New York: Harcourt Brace Jovanovich, 1970.

Davis, Adelle. *Let's Get Well.* New York: Harcourt Brace Jovanovich, 1965.

Davis, Adelle. *Let's Have Healthy Children,* new and exp. ed. New York: Harcourt Brace Jovanovich, 1972.

Davis, Francyne. *Low Blood Sugar Cookbook.* New York: Bantam Books, Inc., 1974.

DiCyan, Erwin. *The Vitamins in Your Life.* New York: Simon and Schuster, 1974.

Duffy, William. *Sugar Blues.* Radnor, Pa.: Chilton Book Co., 1975.

Elwood, Catharyn. *Feel Like a Million.* New York: Pocket Books, Inc., 1976.

Ewald, Ellen B. *Recipes for a Small Planet.* New York: Ballantine Books, Inc., 1975.

Feingold, Ben F. *Why Your Child Is Hyperactive.* New York: Random House Inc., 1974.

Ford, Margie, et al. *The Deaf Smith Country Cookbook: Natural Foods from Family Kitchens.* New York: Macmillan Publishing Co., Inc., 1973.

Fredericks, Carlton. *Eating Right for You.* New York: Grosset and Dunlap, Inc., 1972.

Fredericks, Carlton, and Bailey, Herbert. *Food Facts and Fallacies.* New York: Arc Books, 1968.

Fredericks, Carlton, and Goodman, Herman. *Low Blood Sugar and You.* New York: Grosset and Dunlap, Inc., 1969.

Goodwin, Mary T., and Pollen, Gerry. *Creative Food Experiences for Children.* Washington, D.C.: Center for Science in the Public Interest, 1974.

Hall, Ross H. *Food for Nought: The Decline in Nutrition,* new ed. New York: Harper and Row (Medical Department), 1974.

Hauser, Gayelord. *Mirror, Mirror on the Wall.* Greenwich, Conn.: Farrar, Straus and Giroux, Inc., 1961.

Hawkins, David, and Pauling, Linus, eds. *Orthomolecular Psychiatry: Treatment of Schizophrenia.* San Francisco, Calif.: W. H. Freeman Co., 1973.

Hightower, Jim. *Eat Your Heart Out: How Food Profiteers Victimize the Consumer.* New York: Crown Publishers, Inc., 1975.

Hoffer, Abram, and Osmond, Humphrey. *How to Live with Schizophrenia,* rev. ed. Secaucus, N.J.: University Books, Inc., 1974.

Hunter, Beatrice T. *Beatrice Trum Hunter's Whole-Grain Baking Sampler.* New Canaan, Conn.: Keats Publishing, Inc., 1972.

Hunter, Beatrice T. *Consumer Beware!* New York: Simon and Schuster, Inc., 1972.

Hunter, Beatrice T. *Fact-Book on Food Additives and Your Health.* New Canaan, Conn.: Keats Publishing, Inc., 1972.

Hunter, Beatrice T. *Fact-Book on Yogurt, Kefir and Other Milk Cultures.* New Canaan, Conn.: Keats Publishing, Inc., 1973.

Hunter, Beatrice T., ed. *Food and Your Health.* New Canaan, Conn.: Keats Publishing, Inc., 1974.

Hunter, Beatrice T. *Natural Foods Cookbook.* New York: Simon and Schuster, Inc., 1969.

Hylton, William H. *The Rodale Herb Book: How to Use, Grow and Buy Nature's Miracle Plants.* Emmaus, Pa.: Rodale Press, Inc., 1974.

Jacobson, Michael F. *Don't Bring Home the Bacon.* Washington, D.C.: Center for Science in the Public Interest.

Jacobson, Michael F. *Your Guide to Better Eating.* Washington, D.C.: Center for Science in the Public Interest.

Jarvis, D. C. *Folk Medicine.* Greenwich, Conn.: Fawcett World Library, 1958.

Kenda, Margaret E., and Williams, Phyliss S. *The Natural Baby Food Cookbook.* New York: Avon Books, 1973.

Kugler, Hans J. *Slowing Down the Aging Process.* New York: Pyramid Publications, 1973.

Lager, Mildred, and Jones, Dorothea Van Gundy. *The Soybean Cookbook.* New York: Arc Books, 1968.

Lappe, Francis M. *Diet for a Small Planet.* San Francisco, Calif.: Ballantine Books, Inc., 1975.

Larson, Gena. *Fact-Book on Better Food for Better Babies and Their Families.* New Canaan, Conn.: Keats Publishing, Inc., 1972.

Longgood, William. *The Darkening Land.* New York: Simon and Schuster Inc., 1972.

Mae, Eydie, and Loeffler, Chris. *How I Conquered Cancer Naturally.* Irvine, Calif.: Harvest House Publishers, 1976.

Marine, Gene, and Van Allan, Judith. *Food Pollution: The Violation of Our Inner Ecology.* New York: Holt, Rinehart and Winston, Inc., 1972.

Martin, Clement G. *Low Blood Sugar: The Hidden Menace of Hypoglycemia.* New York: Arc Books, 1974.

Newman, Marcea. *The Sweet Life: Marcea Newman's Natural Food Dessert Cookbook.* New York: Houghton Mifflin Co., 1974.

Nittler, Alan. *A New Breed of Doctor.* New York: Pyramid Books, 1974.

Nusz, Frieda. *The Natural Foods Blender Cookbook.* New Canaan, Conn.: Keats Publishing, Inc., 1972.

Ogden, Samuel. *Step by Step to Organic Vegetable Growing.* Emmaus, Pa.: Rodale Press, Inc., 1971.

Page, Melvin E., and Abrams, H. Leon. *Your Body Is Your Best Doctor.* New Canaan, Conn.: Keats Publishing, Inc., 1972.

Passwater, Richard. *Supernutrition: Megavitamin Revolution.* New York: Dial Press, 1975.

Paterson, Grusha D., Editor. *Health's-a-Poppin'.* New York: Pyramid Books, 1973.

Pauling, Linus. *Vitamin C and the Common Cold.* San Francisco, Calif.: W. H. Freeman Co., 1970.

Pfeiffer, Carl C. *Mental and Elemental Nutrients: A Physicians' Guide to Nutrition and Health Care.* New Canaan, Conn.: Keats Publishing Inc., 1976.

Pinckney, Edward R., and Pinckney, Cathey. *The Cholesterol Controversy.* Los Angeles: Sherbourne Press, 1973.

Pomeroy, L. R., ed. *New Dynamics of Preventive Medicine.* 2 vols. New York: Stratton Intercontinental Medical Books Corp., 1974.

Ratcliff, J. D. *Your Body and How It Works.* Pleasantville, N.Y.: Reader's Digest Press/Delacorte Press, 1975.

Robbins, William. *The American Food Scandal.* New York: William Morrow and Co., Inc., 1974.

Rosenberg, Harold, and Feldzaman, A. N. *The Doctor's Book of Vitamin Therapy.* New York: G. P. Putnam's Sons, 1974.

Schroeder, Henry A. *The Trace Elements and Man.* Old Greenwich, Conn.: The Devin-Adair Co., 1973.

Selye, Hans. *The Stress of Life.* New York: McGraw-Hill, 1956.

Shute, Wilfred E., and Taub, Harald. *Vitamin E for Ailing and Healthy Hearts.* New York: Pyramid Publications, Inc., 1972.

Spira, Ruth R. *Naturally Chinese: Healthful Cooking from China.* Emmaus, Pa.: Rodale Press, Inc., 1974.

Stone, Irwin. *The Healing Factor: Vitamin C Against Disease.* New York: Grosset & Dunlap, 1972.

Suttie, J. W. *Introduction to Biochemistry.* New York: Holt, Rinehart and Winston, 1972.

Taub, Harald J. *Keeping Healthy in a Polluted World.* New York: Harper and Row Publishers, Inc., 1974.

Tobe, John H. *The Natural Foods No-Cookbook.* Don Mills, Ontario: Greywood Publishing Limited, 1973.

Turner, James S. *Chemical Feast: Report on the Food and Drug Administration.* (Ralph Nader Study Group Reports) New York: Grossman Publishers, Inc., 1970.

Verrett, Jacqueline, and Carper, Jean. *Eating May Be Hazardous to Your Health.* New York: Simon and Schuster, Inc., 1974.

Wade, Carlson. *Fact-Book on Fats, Oils and Cholesterol.* New Canaan, Conn.: Keats Publishing, Inc., 1973.

Wallis, Arthur. *God's Chosen Fast.* Fort Washington, Pa.: Christian Literature Crusade, 1970.

Watson, George. *Nutrition and Your Mind: The Psychochemical Response.* New York: Harper and Row, 1972.

Williams, Roger J. *Alcoholism: The Nutritional Approach.* Austin, Tex.: University of Texas Press, 1959.

Williams, Roger J. *Biochemical Individuality: The Basis for the Genetotrophic Concept.* Austin, Tex.: University of Texas Press, 1969.

Williams, Roger J. *Nutrition Against Disease.* New York: Bantam Books, Inc., 1973.

Williams, Roger J. *Nutrition in a Nutshell.* New York: Doubleday, 1962.

Williams, Roger J. *The Wonderful World Within You: Your Inner Nutritional Environment.* New York: Bantam Books, Inc., 1976.

Yudkin, John. *Sweet and Dangerous.* New York: Bantam Books, Inc., 1973.